Patient Education Plus

The Professional Developments Series

These five books provide you with a wealth of insight into all aspects of nursing practice. The series is essential reading for qualified, practising nurses who need to keep up with new developments, evaluate their clinical practice and develop and extend their clinical management and teaching skills. Up-to-date, and appropriately illustrated, The Professional Developments Series brings together the work of well over a hundred nurses.

Other titles in The Professional Developments Series:

The Ward Sister's Survival Guide

This book is essential reading and valuable reference for all nurses with direct clinical management responsibility.

Practice Check!

How well do you communicate with colleagues and patients? How do you respond when difficult situations arise? You can explore your responses to all these – and more – by using this book. Each Practice Check presents brief descriptions of situations which may arise in practice, together with open-ended questions and discussion to enable you to explore the problems and establish your own solutions.

The Staff Nurse's Survival Guide

Relevant to nurses working in all healthcare settings, this brings together chapters on a wide range of clinical and non-clinical issues in patient care, and includes a practical section on looking after *yourself*, too.

Effective Communication

Good communication is an essential aspect of nursing, in every healthcare setting, and this title in the series covers a wide range of topics, including counselling, confidentiality, group and team work, compliance and communicating with children.

These books are available from the publishers:

Austen Cornish Publishers Limited
Brook House
2–16 Torrington Place
London WC1E 7LT
Tel: 071-636 4622

Ask to be included on their mailing list!

Patient Education Plus

A collection of Patient Education Plus articles
first published in The Professional Nurse
and here revised and updated

Austen Cornish Publishers Limited
London
1990

Patient Education Plus
First published in 1990. Reprinted 1990

Austen Cornish Publishers Limited
Brook House
2–16 Torrington Place
London WC1E 7LT

ISBN 1 870065 11 5

Printed and bound in Great Britain by Richard Clay Limited,
Bungay, Suffolk

Contents

Introduction

One of the most significant developments in nursing within the last decade is the acknowledgement by nurses themselves, by other health professionals and by patients and clients that the practice of nursing routinely includes a patient teaching role.

'Teaching' and 'education' are terms which are used in many different ways by different people in different contexts, and this is how this part of your nursing role often is in practice. For one patient, you may need to explain a self-care procedure clearly and simply, to teach them in a direct way how to manage with, for example, a new stoma or a catheter at home. For another patient you may be aware of the value to them of assessing how much they *really* know about diet – for themselves or for their child or partner – and then you may decide to encourage them to find out more for themselves and develop the skills needed to manage diet more effectively. Sometimes the 'teaching' is so informal that you may describe it more accurately as support or guidance.

Whatever the form of teaching, and however long its timescale, you will be using the skills of teaching and assessing knowledge and expertise every day of your working life, whatever the healthcare setting. This book brings together a selection of Patient Education Plus articles which were first published in *The Professional Nurse* magazine, and which have been revised and updated for this collection.

Each chapter looks at a different clinical topic and discusses the likely nature of your teaching role with these patients and clients. Subject matter ranges from healthy life-style issues such as sunbathing, smoking, preventing heart disease, cancer self-examination, minimising Aids risk and planning a diet to more specific teaching and assessment required by clients with chronic conditions, a requirement for self care for example with catheterisation, long-term dietary change and diabetes. Each chapter includes a handout which can be photocopied freely for distribution for patients or clients, or can be adapted to suit particular local policies, or the special needs of individual clients. I hope that you and your colleagues will find that this is a useful source book of ideas and practical help with this vital area of your work.

Elizabeth M Horne,
Editorial Director, The Professional Nurse,
London, November 1989.

Staying Healthy

This Patient Education Plus is intended as a Self-Education Plus – although you could use it with patients too. Elizabeth Horne, with your best interests at heart, asks you to take a good look at your own life style and assess how healthy it really is.

Your healthy life style

Elizabeth M. Horne, MA
Editorial Director, The Professional Nurse

1. We are what we eat!

Keep a Food Diary for 3 days. Make a note of everything you eat and drink in that period, and estimate the total amounts of fats, carbohydrates, proteins, salt and other minerals, fibre, and vitamins that you consume each day. Try and assess the *balance* between these. Also, check your current body weight.

2. How physically fit and well are you?

Assess your level of physical fitness and the activites that could contribute towards this. Are you satisfied? Do you make regular checks on your own health? Do you seek regular medical and dental check-ups?

3. Are you over-using drugs?

Assess your daily average intake of alcohol, tobacco, caffeine, and any other drugs (medicinal or otherwise). Are these levels dangerous to your health, or likely to become so?

4. How do you feel?

Our own mental health must be the hardest part of our health profile to assess for ourselves, because of the difficulty we all have in being objective about our own feelings and emotional needs. Perhaps the questions in this section will set you thinking and reassessing your own needs.

Chart your health profile now and set your goals for the next six months on the grids on the facing page.

If nurses are to have an effective role in health education, should they consider whether the role model that they as individuals represent to their patients and clients is appropriate? Will their health education message be taken seriously?

Define your own health profile by completing the first column of each of the four sections. You will need to set your own standards for each criterion. Decide whether this profile needs improvement, and if you think it does, set yourself some objectives for the next six months. Try and be realistic: there is no limit to the number and range of factors that you can change at any one time, and remember that one single change (such as giving up smoking) will have an effect on *several* parts of your health profile. Don't be too tough on yourself – remember your *mental* health, too! Plan your strategy with a friend or colleague, if this helps.

Useful sources of information

Health Education Council (1984) Looking After Yourself. HEC, London.
  A useful short guide to healthy living.
(1984) Food for Thought. HEC, London.
  Brief advice on nutrition and patterns of eating.
(1985) Guide to a Healthy Sex Life. HEC, London.
  Very brief information on sexually transmitted diseases.
HMSO (1985) Drug Misuse: A Basic Briefing. Institute for the Study of Drug Dependence, London.

A short but detailed guide to drug abuse.
Rogers, C. and Stevens, B. (1967) Person to Person: The Problem of Being Human. Souvenir Press, London.
  A thought-provoking book which may shed some light on maintaining mental health.
Vetter, C. (1979) It's Your Life. Accept Publications, London.
  A short booklet on alcohol abuse.
Ward, L., (1984): Facts about Smoking: A Trainers' Manual. Health Education Council, London.
  A valuable review of research into the effects of smoking.

Alcohol consumption. The amount of alcohol is roughly the same in half a pint of beer or lager, one measure of vermouth or spirits, one glass of wine and one small glass of sherry or port. Using this amount as a "standard" measure, safe limits and health-threatening levels of alcohol consumption can be suggested.

	Safe limits	Levels that threaten health
Men	4·5 standard measures 2 or 3 times a week	8 standard measures a day
Women	2·3 standard drinks 2 or 3 times a week	5 standard measures a day

Recommended daily intake of energy and nutrients for healthy, moderately active adults.

	Average body weight (depends on height)	Energy (kcal)	Fats (preferably unsaturated)	Protein	NaCC	Iron	Ascorbic acid (vitamin C)	Other vitamins and minerals
Men	65g	3,000kcal of which 700 should come from fats	75	75g	1·2g	10mg	750mg	Sufficient vitamins and minerals for a healthy person are normally present in a reasonably balanced diet
Women	55kg	2,000kcal of which 520 should come from fats	56	55g	1·2g	12mg	750mg	

Section 1.	Present health profile					Aim for the next 6 months					Achievement in 6 months				
	Appalling	Poor	Fair	Good	Excellent	Appalling	Poor	Fair	Good	Excellent	Appalling	Poor	Fair	Good	Excellent
Total daily intake of carbohydrate															
Total daily intake of saturated fats															
Total daily salt intake															
Total daily fibre intake															
Total daily intake of vitamins and minerals other than salt															
Balance between nutrients															
Your weight															

Section 2.	Present health profile			Aim for the next 6 months			Achievement in 6 months		
	No	Sometimes	Yes	No	Sometimes	Yes	No	Sometimes	Yes
Do you take some form of daily exercise?									
Is your level of exercise high enough?									
Do you make regular self-health checks. eg breast self-examination/testicular self-examination?									
Do you have regular medical check-ups?									
Do you ignore symptoms of your own ill health?									
Do you visit the dentist regularly?									
Are your feet healthy?									
Is your sex-life healthy?									

Section 3.	Present health profile			Aim for the next 6 months			Achievement in 6 months		
	No	Sometimes	Yes	No	Sometimes	Yes	No	Sometimes	Yes
Alcohol									
Tobacco									
Caffeine									
Other drugs									
Do you mix drugs?									

Section 4.	Present health profile			Aim for the next 6 months			Achievement in 6 months		
	No	Sometimes	Yes	No	Sometimes	Yes	No	Sometimes	Yes
Are you coping with the level of stress you experience?									
Do you experience periods of depression or intense irritability?									
Are you dependent upon a drug or drugs?									
Do you frequently feel lonely or isolated?									
Do you take regular relaxing holidays. and make enough time available for family and friends?									
Do you get enough undisturbed sleep?									

Do nurses have sufficient knowledge about the dangers of over-exposure to the sun to be able to give effective health education?

Out in the mid-day sun?
Nurses' perceptions of the dangers of sun exposure

Patricia Osborne, RGN, DipN
Nurse Tutor, Mid Glamorgan School of Nursing, Merthyr Tydfil

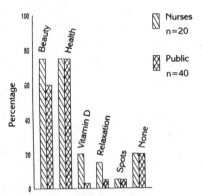

Figure 1. Perceived benefits of sun exposure.

Why do we sunbathe?

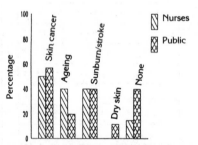

Figure 2. Perceived hazards of sun exposure.

Complexion	Burn and Tan History	Skin Type
Very fair	Always burns; never tans	1
Fair	Burns easily; tans minimally	11
Light to medium	Burns moderately; tans slowly	111
Medium	Burns minimally; always tans	1V
Dark brown	Rarely burns; tans well	V
Black	Never burns; deeply pigmented skin which may or may not darken.	V1

Table 1. Skin type assessment scale (assessment according to complexion and burn and tan history (Greiter, 1982).

Aim of the study

Awareness of the association between the sun and skin cancer has been growing in recent years. The medical profession expressed its concern in a report which highlighted the association (RCP, 1987), while in the same year, the European Commission launched a three year campaign entitled Europe against Cancer. Their report said 40 per cent of Europeans were still unaware of simple cancer prevention, such as stopping smoking and limiting sun exposure (CEC, 1987).

It is now well established that exposure to ultraviolet rays, particularly the UV-B rays, can cause skin cancer, and it has been suggested that 'Celtic' skin types are particularly prone to melanomas (Lane et al, 1973). The incidence of skin cancers, especially melanomas, is doubling every decade and Mackie (1982) says this must be related to the average threefold increase in exposure to the sun over the last decade, perhaps influenced by increased leisure opportunities and the popularity of holidays in the sun.

If sunbathing is so potentially harmful, why do we do it? Because we don't know about the hazards, or because we don't know how to protect ourselves?

Between nine and 15 per cent of the editorial content of women's magazines cover health related topics, and they are a major source of information (White, 1970; Amos, 1985). However much of their advertising and fashion content endorses suntans. While travel features discuss innoculations, the hazards of local drinking water and local medical services, little, if any, mention is made of sun exposure or even heat exposure. Health features which do discuss sun protection may well be inaccurate, especially with regard to the physiology of a sun tan and how to choose an appropriate sun protection factor (SPF), which is designed to filter out harmful sunrays. The SPF number corresponds to the time the user can be exposed to the sun without burning. For example, SPF 6 means, theoretically, a person can stay in the sun six times longer than without any protection.

Travel brochures also make their holidays inviting by concentrating almost entirely on sun, sand and sea. The small print on medical insurance and innoculations makes no mention of sun exposure or protection. Companies producing sun creams and lotions also produce leaflets to accompany their products, but it is clear that the main aim of the leaflets is advertising rather than information. Not all companies appear to make the full range of SPFs (up to factor 15 or even higher), tending to centre around the middle range of 8 – 10.

While it is clear the sun can be harmful, the information made available to the public appears to be inconsistent and at times incomplete. With this in mind it was decided to investigate the extent of registered nurses' knowledge on sun protection and compare it with a sample of non-nurses.

The aim of the study was to answer the question, do nurses have sufficient knowledge to advise and carry out a health education role in relation to sun exposure and protection? It was also intended to compare

Method

1. Does it itch?
2. Is its diameter 1 cm or larger?
3. Is it growing?
4. Is it irregular in shape?
5. Does the density of black and brown colour vary?
6. Is the patch inflamed?
7. Is there crusting and bleeding?

Table 2. Check list for skin examination.

The sample

Results

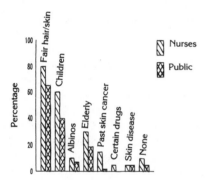

Figure 3. Groups perceived to need specific precautions against UVR.

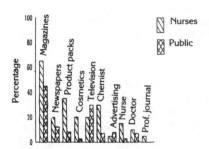

Figure 4. Sources of knowledge and information.

Discussion

their use of SPFs with that of non-nurses, to establish whether their reported use was safer than the non-nurses.

A comparative survey was designed using a structured interview. Five main areas were identified for further development:

Sunbathing habits Did the subject sunbathe? For how long? In what circumstances? Was any kind of protection used?

Sun protection practice Was there any understanding of SPFs? How were they used? How were they applied? When were they applied?

Beliefs and knowledge source Why did the subject sunbathe? How was knowledge gained and habits influenced?

Recognition of potential problems Was self-examination of the skin performed? Could the individual identify suspicious lesions?

Skin type What skin type was the respondent? (Table 1).

Following approval from the nursing ethics committee, a sample of 20 registered nurses and 40 non-nurses were selected. The non-nurses formed an opportunity sample. This non-probability sampling method means the inferences that can be made about the general public are limited. Since there were no indicators as to what size group would be required to form a representative sample, 40 was felt to be sufficient to establish a reasonable pattern.

The proportions within the two groups who admitted to sunbathing were similar – 90 per cent of nurses and 83 per cent of non-nurses. Of these, 10 per cent of the public sample did not use any form of sun protection, while all the nurses claimed to use some form of protection; 50 per cent of the public sample and 80 per cent of nurses used a product containing an SPF. However, in both groups, the choice of factor did not often correspond to the user's skin type, and 50 per cent of the public and 55 per cent of nurses only used an SPF when sunbathing and not at any other time such as walking, sightseeing and playing outdoor sport.

The most commonly considered benefits of sunbathing for both groups were health and beauty (Figure 1), while perceived hazards of sun exposure were again similar, with skin cancer being the most frequently mentioned (Figure 2). It should be noted that 40 per cent of non-nurses and 15 per cent of the nurses did not know of any hazards of sun exposure. The two groups were also asked which types of people they thought require special protection when exposed to the sun, and most cited children and those with fair skin (Figure 3). Magazines were the most common source of knowledge and information, while health professionals and professional journals provide only a minority of knowledge source (Figure 4).

When it came to recognising potential skin problems, particularly suspicious moles, less than half (40 per cent) of the public sample, but all the nurses, could list symptoms of itching, bleeding, soreness, enlargement and pigmentation. The RCP's report (1987) suggests a seven point check list for self-skin examination (Table 2).

In response to the question "If you were told sunbathing could be harmful; would this stop you from sunbathing?" 65 per cent of the public and 70 per cent of nurses said they would **not** stop or alter their sunbathing habits.

While the study was small, several important factors came to light which warrant discussion. The majority of those in the sample sunbathe regularly without taking suitable precautions. Sun protection such as hats and T-shirts, were only used after burning had occurred; "when shoulders start to feel sore".

These people in the study sunbathed in the belief that tanning is healthy and beautiful. Paradoxically, most were aware of the hazards associated with it. Nearly all knew that those with fair skin need to take extra care, and yet a combined total of 70 per cent of the respondents fell

References

Amos, E. (1985) British women's magazines – a healthy read? Health Education in the Media, Pergamon, Oxford.

Commission of the European Communities (1987) Europeans and the prevention of cancer – a public opinion survey. CEC, London.

Jaffe, M. (1987) All white now. *Observer Magazine*, June 14.

Johnson, E.Y. and Lookingbill, D.P. (1984) Sunscreen use and sun exposure. *Archives of Dermatology*, **120**, 6, 727-31.

Lane, A., Brown, M.M., Melia, D.F. (1973) "Celticity" and cutaneous malignant melanoma in Massachusetts. *Pigment Cell*, **1**, 29.

Mackie, R. and Aitchison, T. (1982) Severe sunburn and subsequent risk of primary cutaneous malignant melanoma in Massachusetts. *Pigment Cell*, **1**, 29.

Mackie, R. and Aitchison, T. (1982) Severe sunburn and subsequent risk of primary cutaneous malignant melanoma in Scotland. *British Journal of Cancer*, **46**, 955-60.

Implications for nurses

References (continued)

Marks, R. (1986) Premalignant disease of the epidermis: Some light on neoplasia. *Journal of the Royal College of Physicians of London* **20**, 2, 116-21.

Royal College of Physicians (1987) Links Between Ultraviolet Radiation and Skin Cancer. RCP, London.

Watson, A. (1983) Sunscreen effectiveness: theoretical and practical considerations. *Australian Journal of Dermatology*, **24**, 1, 17-22.

White, C. (1970) Women's Magazines 1693-1963. Michael Joseph, London.

Halting the rise in skin cancers

into this category, and their own protection measures were often inadequate.

It was notable that the most common source of information was magazines. While there is a great deal of health related material in women's magazines, other factors, such as their presentation, advertisements and fashion can be contradictory, and do not always support or propound their articles (the most obvious example being advertisements for cigarettes). It is sad to note that professional journals are not a source of information for nurses. Although little has been written until relatively recently about sun exposure and protection, the evidence is accumulating and becoming more accessible to nurses.

The most concerning statistic in the study is the proportion of participants who would not change their habits even if told of the dangers of excessive sun exposure. This is not a new revelation, as demonstrated by others (Johnson et al, 1984; Watson, 1983). Marks (1986) believes that unless fashions change and brown, tanned skin ceases to be desirable, information will not be enough to influence people. However, there are signs that fashions might dictate change. Rock cult figures have always been exponents of 'un-sunned skin', while top fashion photographers are beginning to prefer untanned models and designers are changing their ideas to support these preferences (Jaffe, 1987).

The nurses in the study demonstrated a lack of knowledge about and poor practice in sun protection. This must be rectified for a number of reasons, not least for the sake of their own health. Active assessment through nursing models and the nursing process allows nurses to observe and act upon any suspicious lesions they may note in their patients, but they can only act if they have the knowledge upon which to do so. Nurses also have a responsibility to set standards and act as role models for others. Some authors (Blum and Robins, 1981) have suggested that if they are to be acceptable and credible role models, their behaviour should conform to safe health practices.

Nurses must be mediators of health education to patients, and this cannot be achieved without the necessary knowledge and expertise. In the past they have been seen only as providers of care and not so much as health educators, this is now changing and knowledge bases must change too. If nurses are to be professionally accountable for their patients' care, they must ensure their knowledge and practice is, and remains, up-to-date.

If the increase in sun related skin diseases, in particular melanomas and non-melanocytic cancers, is to be halted, health education for all members of the public is vital. America and Australia have already developed nationwide campaigns – The Australian slogan 'Slip, Slap, Slop' is particularly apt (slip on a top, slap on a hat, slop on a sunscreen).

Magazines and newspapers, should collaborate with health professionals to ensure accurate reporting about sun exposure. This important partnership is already evident in AIDS education, and must be developed further in other areas. Holiday companies should also consider accepting some responsibility for education and advice by including advice about sun protection in their brochures, while companies who manufacture sunscreens also need to provide accurate and clear information to the consumer.

How Safe is Sunbathing?

If you are planning a holiday in the sun within the next few weeks, give some thought to the powerful and potentially harmful effects of sunlight.

What is a sun tan?

The colour of skin depends on four pigments, one of which is melanin, the dark colour which is produced in response to sunlight. There is no difference in the number of melanocytes between people of different natural skin colour, but the distribution of the pigment in the cells is different, and the rate of production of melanin is higher in dark-skinned people than in fair-skinned people. Melanin protects the skin against sunburn by absorbing ultraviolet (UV) light, so dark-skinned people have more natural protection against the harmful effects of the sun than fair-skinned.

People vary in the rate at which they produce melanin, and for many fair-skinned people, sun tanning is a slow process. For everybody, the rate of production of melanin increases only gradually, and the maximum rate is reached at first by only a limited exposure to UV light. Further exposure to sunlight will cause burning. In strong sunlight, this will happen in untanned and fair skin in 10-15 minutes so it is important to protect the skin with clothes or effective sunscreen preparations.

Effective screening

An effective sun screening agent is zinc oxide, which is an ingredient of some sunscreens although these may be cosmetically unsatisfactory. Otherwise choose sun screening preparations containing para-aminobenzoic acid (PABA). The sunscreen ratings which some manufacturers use to indicate the degree of protection their preparations give are, unfortunately, not part of a standardised measure, so you need to assess the effectiveness of each manufacturer's range. Some preparations are waterproof, others will need reapplying after swimming. All preparations need reapplying approximately every two hours.

If you are in sunlight on a beach, particularly with white sand, or on snow, the effect of sunlight is enhanced because UV light is reflected from water and snow, as well as reaching you directly from the sun. Delicate skin (such as that on the backs of your knees) and the skin of children are particularly vulnerable, and extra care should be taken to protect these.

What are the risks?

Sunburn if your skin is exposed to the sun for too long, you will get sunburn. The skin becomes red and painful (first degree burning) and, if burning continues, may become blistered (second degree burning). Mild first degree burning can be treated with bland creams applied several times a day; cold water compresses or immersion in cold water will, although painful at the time, help to remove heat from the burns

and reduce the burning effect. Milk is an effective treatment for mild sunburn. Medical treatment should be sought for second degree burning.

Sunstroke If your exposure to sunlight is prolonged, sunburn will become severe and you may experience nausea, headaches and fainting. This is sometimes termed 'sunstroke'. If this condition lasts longer than 12 hours, medical help should be sought. Immediate medical treatment is required for children.

Dehydration Everyone, and particularly small children, will become seriously dehydrated in hot weather unless they take a lot of fluid, so keep drinking soft drinks! Dehydration is usually accompanied by headaches and a hangover-like feeling.

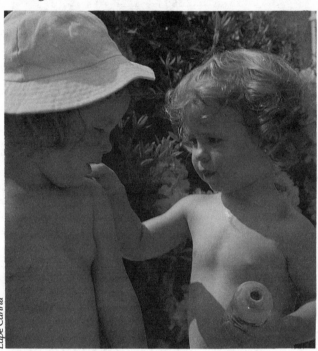

Children need particularly strong sunscreens.

Ageing Exposure to sunlight increases the rate at which the skin visibly ages: dehydration of both skin and hair occur rapidly in hot sunshine, and coarse wrinkles and changes in the skin's tissue develop much more rapidly in people who expose their skin to the sun regularly.

Cancer You increase your risk of developing any of three different forms of skin cancer if you increase your exposure to sunlight. Any skin lesion or colour or texture change in the skin should be taken seriously, as it may indicate that some skin cells have become malignant. Medical attention should be sought immediately if any change takes place in the skin. Some moles are particularly susceptible to this kind of change and intermittent irritation may be the first indication. Skin cancers occur much more frequently in parts of the skin exposed to sunlight than those which are rarely exposed. The incidence of skin cancers in the UK has increased by 8-10 per cent a year with increased overseas holiday travel.

Prickly heat If the outflow of sweat from the skin is obstructed, it builds up within the skin and pinhead-sized blisters appear. This gives an itchy and burning sensation and tends to persist once it has begun. Staying cool, by using air conditioners or fans, and by wearing loose, cool clothing will minimise the problem.

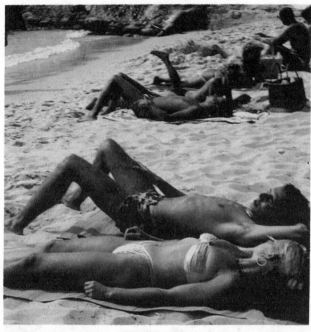

Always use an effective sunscreen when sunbathing.

Risks to your eyes Your eyes are very sensitive and the retina and lens can be damaged by strong light. Wear a hat or good quality sunglasses to screen UV light, and take care when using binoculars, field glasses or

cameras, as reflected light (for example, from water) can be very powerful. Never look directly at the sun with optical instruments; this would rapidly and permanently damage the retina of your eyes.

Are you in contact with or taking any of these? If so take extra care in the sun.	
Ingested chemicals producing photosensitivity:	**Topical (ie, skin-applied)**
Phenothiazines	Bithionol
Tetracyclines	Terachlorosalicylanilide
Sulfonamides	Coal tar preparations
Chlorothiazide	Perfumes
Barbiturates	Laundry whiteners
Chloroquine	Citrus fruits
Quinine	Sap from certain plants, including those in the *Umbelliferae* family
Psoralens	
Sulfonylureas	
Gold	
Oral contraceptives	

Photosensitivity Some skin diseases, and certain chemical agents may increase sensitivity to sunlight. Among the chemical photosensitisers are some perfumes, laundry whiteners, citrus fruit juice (applied to the skin), sap from certain plants and a number of drugs including oral contraceptives, tetracyclines, sulphonomides, phenothiazines and barbiturates (Table 1).

Benefits of sunlight
You may be wondering if exposure to the sun has any value! In moderate doses, and with sensible precautions, sunlight is a beneficial agent in promoting healing of skin conditions such as acne, and in providing a comfortable sense of wellbeing. And a light tan does make you feel good!

Remember the golden rules

● Limit exposure of untanned skin to the sun to 15 minutes on your first day and gradually increase this as your skin's tolerance builds up. This way, you will avoid sunburn and gradually develop a tan. Always avoid direct exposure to the intense sunlight between 10.00am and 3.00pm. Also be careful in the morning and evening as the reflections of ultraviolet light can be more intense than they seem.

● Use a sunscreen preparation to protect exposed skin: use a higher protection preparation at first and remember to reapply this after swimming. Some waterproof sunscreen preparations are available. All preparations need to be reapplied regularly to continue to be effective.

● Use lipscreens to protect your lips.

● Wear a hat or good quality sunglasses to screen UV light and protect your eyes.

● Ultraviolet light can still reach you through an overcast sky, so take the same precautions on lightly cloudy days in hotter countries.

● Children are particularly vulnerable to both sunburn and dehydration.

● Don't use perfume when in the sun and remember that some drugs may make your skin even more sensitive to sunlight.

● Take any change in the colour, texture or size of moles or other areas of your skin seriously and see a doctor straight away.

How many more smokers can be encouraged to kick the habit, which is now widely known to be a health hazard? There are currently eight million ex-smokers in the UK. Nurses have a key role in helping patients to give up but with over half the profession still smoking, are we setting patients the best example? Here are some practical suggestions to help all those who want to stop smoking.

Stop smoking!
Practical ideas for nurses and patients

Sally Kendall, BSc, RGN, NV
Lecturer in Nursing at Buckinghamshire College of Higher Education

With the increasing number of articles and reports in newspapers and magazines and on television and radio, most smokers will probably be aware of the health-threatening effects of their habit, on themselves and on those non-smokers who live or work in the same environment. The anti-smoking lobby has become more articulate, and concern over the dangers of tobacco smoke have lead to increasing restrictions on smoking in many public places. But giving up smoking isn't easy, and most smokers will need the support of their friends and family. This Patient Education Plus will provide a starting point.

As a nurse you should familiarize yourself with the physiological and pathological effects of smoking. Many smokers know that smoking is bad for them, but few are fully aware of all the facts. You should be prepared to give such information if and when it seems appropriate. On average, people who smoke lose 10-15 years of their life. Among 1,000 men who smoke, about six will be killed on the roads, but 250 will be killed before their time by tobacco. About six out of 10 smokers say that they would like to stop. If any of your patients, clients, or friends would like to give up smoking it may be useful to go through the suggestions on the handout sheet with them. Fill in the name of a contact for the patient and tell them how they can contact them.

It may be useful for nurses to find out the following information:

Is there a District smoking policy?
If so, how does it affect patients/clients smoking on health services premises? How could you make use of this in your advice to smokers?

Is there a smokers' clinic in your District?
If so, how are referrals made? Is it a walk-in clinic or not?

Is nicotine chewing gum available from GPs in your District?
It will only be available on private prescription but it is worth finding out whether GPs are willing to prescribe it at all before sending patients off to their doctor to ask for it!

Further reading (for patients, clients and yourself) and useful addresses

ASH (1985) Smoking Prevention – a Health Promotion Guide for the NHS. An ASH (Action on Smoking and Health) handbook, London.
Health Education Authority (1989) Smoking Resource Pack, HEA, London.
Health Education Council (1984) *So You Want To Stop Smoking* HEC, London.
Stoppard, M. (1985) *Quit Smoking*. BBC Publications, London.
Royal College of Physicians (1983) Health or Smoking? A Report of the Royal College of Physicians. Pitman Medical, London.

Useful Addresses
ASH (Action on Smoking and Health), Margaret Pyke House, 5-11 Mortimer Street, London W1N 7RH.
Health Education Authority, Hamilton House, Mabledon Place, London WC1H 9TX.
Scottish Health Education Group, Woodburn House, Canaan Lane, Edinburgh EH10 4SG.

ASK YOUR NURSE ABOUT HOW TO
STOP
SMOKING

- Think about how much you want to give up smoking, how determined you are to stop, and how sure you are that you will succeed. Be honest with yourself! If the answer to all three is ''very much'' then you are well on the way.

- Think about the things that really worry you about smoking. It may be the effect on your own health or that of your family or baby. You may be more concerned about the cost. List your worries here:

  ....

  ....

  ....

  ....

  ....

- Think about the things that will improve when you give up smoking. List them here:

  ....

  ....

  ....

  ....

  ....

- How are you going to manage when you are craving for a cigarette? Some people find nibbling helpful (try to stick to fruit, raw vegetables, or chewing gum). Others find it useful to avoid habits such as smoking with coffee, after dinner, or while on the telephone. By changing your routine you can avoid situations in which you know you will have a strong urge to smoke. Think about *your* daily routine and write down here ways that will help you to overcome the craving:

  ....

  ....

  ....

  ....

  ....

- Take it one day at a time — you have just made a big change in your life.

- Make a plan for yourself. The evidence shows that deciding on a day to stop completely is more successful than stopping gradually. Some people find it useful to tell other people about their plan; make a ''contract'' to stop, or a bet, or get someone to sponsor you if it will help. Prepare for the day by getting rid of cigarettes, lighters and ashtrays and just stop completely on the day that you have chosen. Write down the date you intend to stop smoking:

  ....

- You may feel irritable when you first give up smoking. Think of ways to relax other than having a cigarette — some people find breathing exercises or gardening helpful. Think about your *own* life style and write down the ways that you are going to cope with irritability:

  ....

  ....

  ....

  ....

  ....

- Try to avoid places where people tend to smoke, such as pubs, and remember that it's all right to say ''No''! Learn to say ''no'' when you are in a tempting situation. Write down the situations that are going to be most difficult for you:

  ....

  ....

  ....

  ....

  ....

- Use this sheet as a reminder. Read over your notes and really think about them. No one is saying that giving up smoking is easy, and some people find it harder than others. You may find that you need some extra support to keep you going. Your nurse, midwife, health visitor, or GP can support you and give you information about smoking and health and the availability in your area of options such as a smokers' clinic. Finally, if you do give in and have a cigarette don't see this as a failing — 8 million people in Britain have stopped smoking so you can too!

- Your contact if you need further support or information is:

  ....

If pregnant women are to be helped to make decisons in the light of their growing demand for non-invasive obstetric techniques, they must understand the reasons behind antenatal procedures and feel confident about asking carers for information.

Antenatal screening

Gill Hooper, SRN, SCM, *Relief Midwife with Southmead Health Authority, Bristol*

Gill Garrett, BA, SRN, RCNT, DN, Cert.Ed(FE), RNT FPCert *Freelance Lecturer, Bristol*

Recent media presentations have portrayed obstetric and midwifery care as polarised into 'high tech' and 'low tech' camps, and the choices within them as being made on solely ideological grounds. Such simplistic portrayals may be very detrimental to the public's perception of the services offered and are very often far removed from reality.

The overall aim of antenatal care is the optimum wellbeing of the mother and her baby. The presence of certain factors are known to render women 'at risk' in pregnancy (Table 1), and sophisticated diagnostic and therapeutic techniques are justified in these cases. For others they may not only be unjustifiably costly, but also unnecessary and intrusive. If the care given is to be appropriate to the pregnant woman's needs, a thorough and sensitive individual assessment must be made, to distinguish between those with actual or potential problems and those likely to remain problem free.

Self determination

Perhaps in no other branch of care is the recognition of the right to self determination so important. While professionals may explain and advise, the pregnant woman and her partner must have the maximum autonomy in decision making. They can only make informed decisions, however, when they have the necessary facts to hand, and it is the duty of all health care professionals to make these available to their clients and to support them through the procedures or investigations subsequently accepted. Without this information, clients may feel pressurised into care they do not want because they do not appreciate its necessity, or they may feel entitled to unnecessary testing which could be actively injurious in their particular circumstances.

As well as using the available clinical methods of screening, assessment of the social and emotional wellbeing of the mother may make a significant contribution to the success of the pregnancy and the birth of a healthy baby. Factors such as nutritional status, dependency on or use of drugs (including tobacco and alcohol), poor relationship with partner, and stress can be sensitively explored in conversation with the mother, and strategies discussed to improve these.

A straightforward account of what antenatal care and testing entails and why, coupled with opportunities for questioning and discussion, and direction towards further information as requested, is a basic prerequisite in care. The handout overleaf has been designed with this in mind and can be photocopied for distribution or adapted to meet local needs.

Table 1. Women generally considered at risk:

The socially deprived.
Those with a history of problems in pregnancy, eg hydramnios, hypertension.
Those with a pre-existing medical condition, eg diabetes.
Those having a previous pregnancy resulting in a handicapped infant.
The obstetrically very young and elderly, ie under 18/over 37.
Women who smoke, drink or take other drugs.
Women of poor nutritional status, eg those with anorexia nervosa.

Antenatal Care – You and Your Baby

During your pregnancy your care may be based at your local maternity hospital, undertaken by your own General Practitioner, 'shared' between the GP and a hospital consultant or, more rarely, supervised by a midwife with hospital backing. Whichever option is chosen, you will be offered comprehensive antenatal care and invited to attend clinics throughout your pregnancy.

Antenatal Routine

Suggested appointments are for the initial 'booking' visit once pregnancy is confirmed (usually at eight to 10 weeks), then monthly between weeks 12 and 28, followed by fortnightly until 36 weeks and then every week until your baby is born. Your partner or a friend may like to come to the clinic with you and would be very welcome.

Antenatal care aims to ensure that you remain healthy and to observe the growth and development of your baby; regular visits help to allow early detection and treatment of any problems which may arise and affect either of you.

The Booking Visit

This visit gives you the opportunity of getting to know the people who will be caring for you and allows them to get to know you.

You will be asked about your personal health and lifestyle (for example, about your eating and smoking habits) and about your family background, in order that any factors which may affect your pregnancy can be noted (for example, the presence of diabetes). You will be weighed, your blood pressure recorded and urine and blood samples will be taken; the results of these tests then form a 'baseline' for comparison with tests on later visits. Any questions you may have about your pregnancy and care can be discussed at this visit and any problems can be dealt with. Information about maternity benefits will be given to you.

Tests on Subsequent Visits

On each visit you will be weighed; your weight gain gives an indication of your baby's growth and development. There are recommended guidelines for weight gain during pregnancy and your midwife will discuss these with you. You will be asked to provide a sample of urine on every attendance which will be tested for the presence of glucose, protein or blood to eliminate the possibility of infection or other problems. Your blood pressure will also be noted to allow early detection of any untoward rise.

To check your growth in relation to the duration of your pregnancy on each visit your abdomen will be felt. In later weeks this examination will tell the doctor or midwife about the position of your baby as the time nears for its birth. A stethoscope will be used to listen to the baby's heartbeat and you will be asked about the baby's movements.

Blood samples will be taken at different stages of your pregnancy. One important test checks that you are not developing anaemia because of your baby's demands on you for iron. Another, which you will be offered at about 16 to 18 weeks is to detect the spinal deformity known as spina bifida in your baby; if this blood test is positive you will be offered further testing and advice.

Ultrasound Scanning

Many women are now offered ultrasound scanning at their local Maternity Hospital, often at around 16 weeks. This 'sound wave' test allows the actual size of your baby to be measured and confirms your expected date of delivery; it also shows where the placenta (afterbirth) lies and can help to detect abnormalities. If problems arise during your pregnancy, further scans can help to indicate what is happening and to assess your baby's development.

Special Tests

If you have had problems with a pregnancy in the past or if you are an older mother or one with known health problems, you may be offered special tests to check on the wellbeing of your baby. These are only carried out when necessary, as they do in themselves carry some risk (such as the very small chance of provoking a miscarriage); and will be discussed very thoroughly with you and your partner should they be felt to be required.

Amniocentesis which is usually done at about 16 to 18 weeks, involves taking a sample of the fluid from around your baby through a needle put in through your abdominal wall. Examination of the fluid can detect spina bifida and chromosome abnormalities such as Downs syndrome; it will also tell the sex of your baby, which is useful if you have a family history of certain sex-linked disorders. Unfortunately some test results can take up to a few weeks to come through and this can be an anxious time for parents.

A newer test used in some areas is, **chorion biopsy** which involves taking a fragment of tissue from around your baby and is carried out through the vagina at about eight to 10 weeks. The results are available more quickly than after an amniocentesis but the test does carry a rather higher risk of miscarriage.

If these tests should show that your baby is handicapped, the doctors will offer to end your pregnancy. You will be given every opportunity to talk things over with the staff caring for you, who will help all they can at this difficult time.

Your Cooperation Card

The results of all your tests will be recorded on the *Cooperation Card* which will be given to you on your booking visit. You keep this card and take it with you to any clinic or hospital appointment. It helps to ensure continuity of care whoever you see during your visits.

News of successful heart or liver transplants is frequently covered by the media, and public awareness may prompt more people to carry donor cards. They may seek advice, or want to discuss their views with a trusted health professional. This article may help you to support them in deciding whether to sign and carry a card.

Donor cards

Celia Wight, SRN, HV Cert
Regional Transplant Coordinator for the East Anglian Health Authority

How often have you been asked about donor cards by a patient, client, patient's relative, or your own family, friends or neighbours? Were they concerned about what it really means to sign and carry one? You may be in a position to encourage these people to consider signing a card. Do you carry one yourself? You probably have your own views on organ donation, and will have decided whether or not you are willing for your own organs to be used to give the opportunity for life or sight to someone else, in the event of an accident or intracranial haemorrhage resulting in brain stem death. Untimely and sudden death isn't an easy topic for anyone to discuss, and it isn't something upon which most people want to dwell. The handout overleaf may provide some answers to questions people often raise in relation to organ donation, and it may form the basis for a discussion. It can be photocopied freely for distribution to clients, patients, relatives and others.

Rising success rates

The number of heart, lung, liver, kidney and corneal transplant operations undertaken in the UK is increasing each year, and the success rates for each are also rising. With the increased availability of transplant surgery, and the higher change of significantly improved life expectancy and quality of life for the recipient, the waiting lists for the different organs are lengthening. Table 1 give some thought provoking statistics about organ transplantation in the UK, and highlights the need for more suitable donors to be identified.

Donor cards for display in your ward, unit or practice can be obtained from: DH (Leaflets), Freepost, Stanmore, Middlesex HA7 1ZZ.

Useful Address
Celia Wight, Chairman
UK Transplant Coordinators Association
Department of Surgery
Addenbrookes Hospital
Hills Road
Cambridge CB2 2QQ

Organ	No. of transplants in 1979	in 1988	Survival rates of recipients in 1979	Survival rates of recipients since 1984	No. of potential recipients on waiting list in January 1989
Heart/ Heart/Lung/ Lung	N/A	340	N/A	80% first year 72% fifth year	419
Liver	12	218	45-50%	73%	157
Kidneys	851	1612	60%	85% (1 year)	3684
Cornea (Tissue typed)	N/A	1131	N/A	N/A 85% of grafts were successful	414

There were an estimated 4,000 cases of brain stem death in the UK in 1985, of which 667 were identified as donors.

Table 1. Number of transplant operations and survival rates in the UK, 1979-1988.

Donor Cards: The Gift of Life

This handout has been prepared to help those who may be seeking guidance and understanding in regard to organ donation.

Will everything possible be done to save life?
Everything medically possible has and will continue to be done for you or your loved one. Doctors who are not responsible for transplantation pronounce death only after established medical criteria have been met and it has been absolutely determined that there is no hope of recovery.

How long must the respirator be kept on after death?
Machine ventilation will continue until the organs can be surgically removed. Without the respirator, oxygenated blood could not reach the organs and they would not be transplantable. The decision to discontinue machine ventilation will be made independently, whether or not the organs are to be donated.

What do the major religious groups say about transplantation?
You are encouraged to talk to your religious adviser if you need guidance. The leading members of all religious groups support organ donation on the basis that this act is essentially a gift of life to another.

Will the funeral be delayed?
Every effort will be made to ensure that there is no unnecessary delay in making funeral arrangements.

Is the body disfigured by organ donation?
No. The operation is carried out under standard sterile conditions in an operating theatre by a full surgical team. The body is treated with respect and reverence.

What will happen after the organs have been removed?
The same procedure will be followed as with any person who dies in hospital. If you wish to see the body after surgery, you have only to consult with your doctor or the nurse in charge who will make appropriate arrangements.

Who will receive the organs?
Recipients are determined by blood group and if necessary by tissue characteristics without regard to sex, race or creed.

Who can be an organ donor?
Anyone, male or female, of any age, of any race, can donate his or her organs. A transplant team will assess the medical suitability of donated organs when the time comes to use them, after the donor's death.

How will you know who the recipients are and if the transplants are successful?
It is not standard practice to divulge names and addresses. Hospital personnel are notified in writing as to where the organs were transplanted.

If you wish you will be given this general information.

Why should I carry a donor card?
It is the best way of ensuring that your wishes are known and followed without confusion or delay if the time comes. Your relatives or close friends will be asked, too, and it may help them to know what your wishes are. It may be helpful to discuss your views with your family and close friends — and they may also wish to carry donor cards, or may already do so.

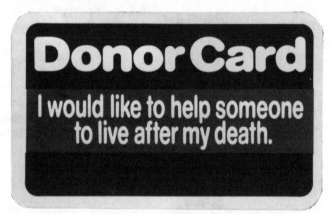

Is it fair to ask the family to make a decision at this tragic and stressful time?
Overwhelming feelings of grief, shock, disbelief and anger are felt by families and friends at a time like this. Yet to be of help in saving lives, organs must be removed shortly after death. The family usually represent what they believe to be the wishes of their loved one.

Have I made the right decision?
Any decision you make is the right one. Organ donation after death can be a gift of life and this charitable act may be a source of comfort in a tragic bereavement. It is important that you feel comfortable and confident in your choice.

Where can I get a donor card?
Donor cards are normally available from your GP's waiting room, a hospital waiting room, or the nurse who gave you this handout.

Alternatively write to: DH (Leaflets), Freepost, Stanmore, Middlesex HA7 1ZZ.

This handout was adapted from the leaflet "A Gift of Life" with kind permission from the UK Transplant Coordinators Association.

Breast screening is a well recognised preventive health measure, yet fear of cancer, or of mutilating surgery, prevents many women from attending clinics.

Breast cancer screening:
Women's reluctance to attend

Patricia A. Black, BA (Hons), RGN
Nurses at the Broad Green Community Unit, Croydon Health Authority

Mass screening of the population at risk (Table 1) undoubtedly improves survival chances for breast cancer sufferers by detecting early tumours, as Adami's study in Sweden (1986) indicates. But any screening programme is only as effective as the number of people who participate in it. A study of individuals who accept or reject screening procedures showed that women were more likely to attend if personally invited, but even if invited only 57.3 per cent did so (Hobbs et al, 1980).

Fear is one possible reason for low participation, but fear of what? Of cancer itself or of the mutilating surgery that may be carried out to cure it? In western culture, the breast has special sexual significance and its removal has a tremendous psychological effect, exceeding the 'normal' period of mourning which follows loss of a body part (Rosen, 1950).

A screening programme must press home the fact that cancer is curable if detected at an early stage. It must include information on new techniques and be aimed at the general population and health professionals.

Lumpectomy, with or without radiotherapy, is a viable alternative in many instances, but women are often justifiably afraid that breast amputation will be the only alternative offered. Some may consider this to be at least as bad as the disease itself. According to Gazet et al (1985) almost three-quarters of British surgeons still opt for mastectomy as the treatment of choice for 75-100 per cent of their patients, as it gives a low rate of recurrence. However, as Harris (1984) and Pickren (1984) point out, breast conservation has a similarly favourable prognosis.

Most breast conservation techniques are carried out in major breast cancer treatment centres. It seems probable that lack of knowledge about new techniques on the part of health care professionals outside these centres is one reason for this; with lack of specialist radiotherapy equipment being another. If health care professionals and women at risk become aware of treatment alternatives they can create a 'demand' for equipment. Health authorities may be reluctant to invest in expensive equipment, but it can be proved cost effective in the long term.

Women might be motivated to attend clinics and overcome fear of disfigurement if services other than breast screening were offered. The concept of 'Well Woman Clinics' could be enlarged to include cervical and coronary heart disease screening as well as counsellors to assist women to come to terms with unfavourable test results.

Information about alternative treatments for early detected breast cancers could be provided, reducing the perceived inevitability of mutilating surgery. More women may then be persuaded to attend clinics.

Morris (1979) has shown that the incidence of psychological morbidity is higher if a woman is not allowed time to adjust to breast loss. To minimise the possibility of psychological disturbance when mastectomy is unavoidable, counselling throughout all stages from diagnosis onwards for both the woman and her partner is crucial. Further, the practice of carrying out mastectomy immediately after a positive 'frozen section' biopsy should be abolished unless exceptional medical circumstances dictate otherwise, as this does not allow the vital adjustment period.

- Early menarche.
- Late age at first pregnancy.
- Nulliparity.
- Upper social class.
- Previous history of benign breast disease.
- Family history of breast cancer.
- Abnormality in steroid metabolism resulting in outputs of C 19 urinary steroids.

Table 1. Women at risk.

Screening programme

In saying that most breast lumps are not malignant, health care professionals must be aware that there are two ways a person may react. If a woman finds a lump in her breast she may be encouraged to attend a clinic to have it investigated as the chances are that it is benign; but on the other hand she may reason that if the chances are that it is benign then why bother to attend clinic in the first place?

References
Adami, H.O. et al (1986) Temporal trends in breast cancer survival in Sweden: significant improvement in 20 years. *JNCI*, **76**, 653-9.
Gazet, J.C., Rainsbury, R.M., Ford, H.T., Powles, T.J. and Coombes, R.C. (1985) Survey of treatment of primary breast cancer in Great Britain. *British Medical Journal*, **290**, 6484, 1793-5.
Harris, J.R. et al (1984) Time, course and prognosis of local recurrence following primary radiation therapy for early breast cancer. *Journal Clin. Oncol.* **2**, 1, 37-41.
Hobbs, P. et al (1980) Acceptors and rejectors of an invitation to undergo breast screening compared with those who referred themselves. *Journal of Epidemiology and Community Health* **34**, 19-22.
Morris, T. (1979) Psychological adjustment to mastectomy. *Cancer Treatment Reviews*, **6**, 41-61.
Pickren, J.W. (1984) Lumpectomy for mammary carcinoma: a retrospective analysis of 40 presumptive candidates from a surgical series. *Cancer*, **15**, 54, 8, 1692-5.
Rosen, V.H. (1950) The role of denial in acute postoperative affective reactions following removal of body parts. *Psychosom. Med.*, **12**, 356.

A Guide to Examining Your Breasts

If you find a lump or anything unusual in your breast, it isn't likely to be serious.

But if it is, the earlier you find it, the easier the cure.

The treatment options now available if it is breast cancer are:

- lumpectomy;

- mastectomy;

- chemotherapy;

- radiotherapy.

Sometimes a combination of these is used. Chemotherapy — the use of drugs to attack the cancer — is not usually used for periods of more than six months.

Mastectomy is more likely to be necessary if the lump is large, which is why screening is so important. Small lumps may only need lumpectomy — removal of just the lump and surrounding tissue — with or without radiotherapy, or possibly only chemotherapy, so the sooner they are detected the more likely you are to keep your breast.

Reconstruction

If a mastectomy is suggested, you may want to discuss the possibility of breast reconstruction. This uses grafts of skin and muscle with the insertion of a silicon implant to rebuild the breast.

It is in your interest to examine your breasts monthly as shown below, especially if you are in an increased risk category.

Increased Risk Categories

1. Family history of breast cancer.

2. Childlessness.

3. First pregnancy at 35+.

4. Periods beginning before age 12 years.

It's important

It takes very little time each month to check for yourself that your breasts are healthy. It's a simple and easy routine and it's important to make it a habit.

By examining your breasts regularly, you get to know what is normal for you. Then you'll find it easy to spot any changes.

If you do find something wrong, you'll be able to get treatment early. In most cases it won't be cancer but just a cyst or growth which can be dealt with very easily, especially when it's found early.

If it is cancer, then early treatment gives you the best chance of a complete cure.

When to examine your breasts

The best time to examine your breasts is just after a period, when your breasts are usually softest and no longer tender. Or, if you've stopped having periods, choose a day in the month you'll be able to remember, like the first day or the last. The important thing is to examine your breasts regularly, at the same time each month.

There are two stages to examining your breasts. The first is looking and the second is feeling.

Looking

When you examine your breasts you're looking for anything that's unusual. For this, looking is just as important as feeling.

Undress to the waist and sit or stand in front of a mirror in a good light. When you look at your breasts, remember that no two are the same — not even your own two. One will probably be slightly larger than the other, and one a little lower on the chest.

Here's what to look for:

- **any change in the size of either breast;**

- **any change in either nipple;**

- **bleeding or discharge from either nipple;**

- **any unusual dimple or puckering on the breast or nipple;**

- **veins standing out more than is usual for you.**

1. First let your arms hang loosely by your sides and look at your breasts in the mirror.

2. Next raise your arms above your head. Watch in the mirror as you turn from side to side to see your breasts from different angles.

3. Now look down at your breasts and squeeze each nipple gently to check for any bleeding or discharge that's unusual for you.

Remember
- If you do find a lump, it is most likely to be harmless.
- If it is cancerous, the quicker it is diagnosed, the more likely you are to keep your breast.

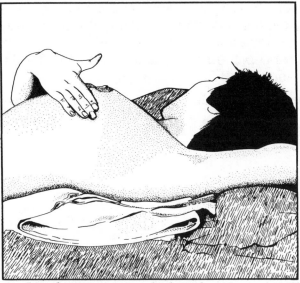

4. Lie down on your bed and make yourself comfortable with your head on a pillow. Examine one breast at a time.

   Put a folded towel under your shoulder-blade on the side you are examining. This helps to spread the breast tissue so that it is easier to examine. Use your right hand to examine your left breast and vice versa. Put the hand you're not using under your head.

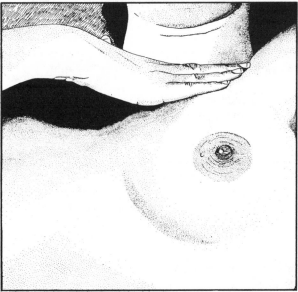

5. Keep your fingers together and use the flat of the fingers, not the tips.

   Start from the collarbone above your breast.

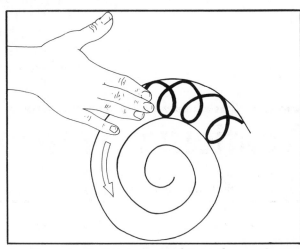

6. Trace a continuous spiral round your breast moving your fingers in small circles. Feel gently but firmly for any unusual lump or thickening.

   Work right round the outside of your breast first. When you get back to your starting point, work round again in a slightly smaller circle, and so on. Keep on doing this until you have worked right up to the nipple. Make sure you cover every part of your breast.

   You may find a ridge of firm tissue in a half-moon shape under your breast. This is quite normal. It is tissue that develops to help support your breast.

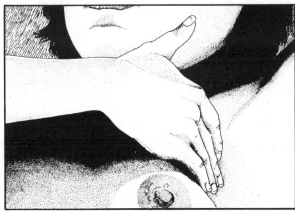

7. Finally, examine your armpit. Still use the flat of your fingers and the same small circular movements to feel for any lumps. Start right up in the hollow of your armpit and gradually work your way down towards your breast. It's important not to forget this last part of the examination.

Any problems?

If you think you've found something unusual in one breast but you're not sure, check the same part of the other breast. If both breasts feel the same, it's probably just the way your breasts are made.

If you still think something may be wrong, then see your doctor. It doesn't matter how uncertain you are. It's far better to see your doctor and set your mind at rest than risk neglecting something serious.

Make a note of where the lump or change is.

Arrange to see your doctor within the next few days. In the meantime, try not to keep feeling the lump to see if it has gone away or got any bigger. It's best to leave it alone.

Adapted from A Guide to Examining Your Breasts, with kind permission of the Health Education Authority.

If you would like advice about examining your breasts, ask your doctor, or the nurse or health visitor at your local clinic.

Testicular self-examination is an effective self-screening procedure that is easily taught, learnt, and practised. It is important for early cancer detection in men in the same way that breast self-examination is for women, and more emphasis needs to be placed on teaching men this health maintenance technique.

Testicular self-examination

James Stanford, BA, RGN, NDN
District Nurse, Brighton Community Nursing Service

Testicular cancer

Testicular cancer was very rare at the beginning of this century, with fewer than 60 deaths a year. However, today approximately one man in 500 will develop testical cancer before he reaches 50. This is the most common solid tumour in men aged 15-35. Although its aetiology is unknown, two factors seem to be related to its incidence:

- **Cryptorchism** Late descended and undescended testes produce an increased risk of developing testicular cancer. If the testes fail to descend or descend after the age of 6, the chance of developing testicular cancer is 11 — 15 per cent.
- **Age** Testicular cancer is the most common solid tumour in men aged 15 — 34, and in America it accounts for 19 per cent of male cancer deaths in this age range.
- **Trauma and infection** These have both been suggested as causative factors, but in each case there is no established link.

Treatment and detection

Over recent years the prognosis for men with testicular tumours has greatly improved. The cure rate is now close to 100 per cent for patients who are identified and treated at an early stage. Even when the cancer has metastasized, cure rates of 60 per cent have been achieved. It is of great importance that the disease is recognized and treated at as early a stage as possible, since any delay in diagnosis will worsen the prognosis. All men can help in the early detection of the disease by performing a simple self-examination procedure.

The awareness of most men regarding testicular cancer and testicular self-examination is somewhat lacking. Unfortunately, it would appear from a survey conducted at one Sussex hospital (Stanford, 1985) that the knowledge base of many nurses is also incomplete. About one half of the nurses were unable to identify those men at high risk of developing the disease. Only half of the female nurses, but nearly 90 per cent of male nurses, knew of testicular self-examination, and while nearly two thirds of the nurses saw the teaching of it as part of their function as health educators, very few had actually taught it to a patient.

The reason for the lack of knowledge of testicular self-examination among the public and among nurses would seem to be a combination of several factors. These include a dearth of educational material in this country, the potential embarrassment that the subject causes many people, and a lack of acceptance by some nurses of their function as health educators. It is to be hoped that more nurses will accept their responsibilities as health educators and help increase their patients' awareness of the importance of self-screening.

Reference
Stanford, J.R. (1987) Testicular self-examination: teaching, learning and practice by nurses. Journal of Advanced Nursing, 12: 1, 13–19.

Bibliography
Cavanaugh, Jr, R.M. (1983) Genital self-examination in adolescent males. *American Family Physician*, 28; 3, 199.
Cummings, K., Metd. (1983) What young men know about testicular cancer. *Preventative Medicine*, 12, 326.
Marty, P.J., and McDermott, R.J. (1983) Teaching about testicular cancer and testicular self-examination. *Journal of School Health*, 53; 6, 351.

TESTICULAR SELF-EXAMINATION

Cancer of the testes is one of the most common cancers in young men. Men who have a history of an undescended or partially descended testicle are at a much higher risk of developing testicular cancer than others.

It takes a while to become confident in doing a self-examination. However, after a time you will become familiar with your own anatomy and will be able to identify any abnormal change. If you find any hard lumps, nodules, or anything that concerns you, you should see your doctor promptly.

Symptoms

The first sign of testicular cancer is often a slight enlargement of one of the testicles and a change in its consistency. There is not normally any pain felt, but there is often a dull ache and a feeling of dragging and heaviness in the groin.

Treatment

The earlier the disease is detected, the better the chance of cure. If treated early, the survival rate is close to 100 per cent. The treatment given varies, but usually includes chemotherapy often combined with surgery and radiation.

Self-examination

- The best way of detecting testicular cancer at an early stage is by a simple monthly self-examination.
- The best time is after a warm bath or shower when the scrotal skin is relaxed (Figure 1).
- Roll each testicle gently between the thumb and fingers of both hands. Your index finger and middle fingers should be on the underside of each testicle and your thumb on top (Figure 2).
- Look and feel for any deviations from normal, especially any hard, small lumps. A normal testicle is ovoid in shape; it should feel firm but not hard and be smooth with no lumps.
- Feel the epididymis, a storage tube that lies behind each testicle. This should feel soft and perhaps slightly tender.
- Feel the spermatic cords which lead upwards from the epididymis and behind the testicles. They should be firm, smooth tubes.

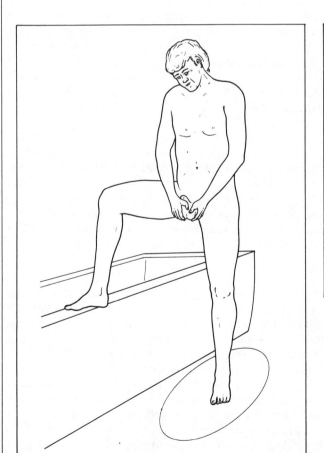

Figure 1. The best time for testicular self-examination is after a warm bath or shower when the scrotal skin is relaxed.

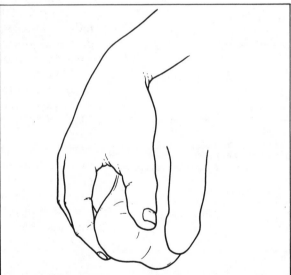

Figure 2. In self-examination, roll each testicle gently between the thumb and fingers to feel for any deviation from normal.

With early detection and treatment, the cure rate for testicular cancer can be up to 100 per cent. That's the incentive for nurses to increase public awareness of the disease and encourage self-examination.

Teaching testicular self-examination

Bettina Schäufele, RGN
Currently working as an agency nurse in London, while studying courses in family planning and holistic medicine

Testicular cancer is a relatively rare disease, representing only about one per cent of all cancers diagnosed in men. However, it is the leading cause of death from cancer in males between the age of 15 to 35 years (Blesch, 1986; Carlin, 1986).

In the early stage of the disease the man might notice a painless enlargement of the testicle, complain of a vague 'heaviness' and he might feel a hard, small lump on palpation. Pain is only present at the later stage, when nerves have been infiltrated as the cancer has metastasised to the lymph nodes or bones. The absence of pain initially, combined with a lack of knowledge, often causes men to delay in seeking medical advice (see Table 1).

Provided the cancer is detected and treated at an early stage, the cure rate is up to 100 per cent, which represents one of the success stories of today's oncology (Davies, 1981). Abnormalities of the testicle can be detected effectively by a regular palpation of the scrotum, yet only a small proportion of the male population have heard of testicular self-examination (TSE) and even fewer practise it regularly. A study conducted in Ireland in 1986 involving 500 men of high socioeconomic and educational status showed that 93 per cent of them were unaware that testicular cancer is a common malignancy between the ages of 15 and 40; testicular self-examination was unknown to 92 per cent of the men. Yet 90 per cent of the men said that they would be interested in more information about cancer of the testis and self-examination (Thornhill et al, 1986). The outcome of the study suggests that either the health care team has not assessed men's health education needs and is not providing adequate information, or that the health education message is not reaching the male population.

Cryptorchidism (undescended testicles).
Family history of testicular cancer.
Previous history of testicular cancer.
Caucasian race.
Possibly trauma.

Table 1. Increased risk factors for testicular cancer.

The nurse's role

As testicular cancer occurs mainly in young men in the prime of their professional life and probably with young, dependent families, the effects of this disease can have an enormous economic, social and emotional impact. How can nurses increase public awareness of testicular cancer and promote regular self-examination? First, as members of the health care profession, nurses need to look at their own attitudes towards health education. They have to accept their responsibility as health educators and need to maintain an up-to-date knowledge (as laid down in the code of professional conduct by the UKCC). Nurses should also regularly assess and evaluate the effectiveness of their communication skills and be aware of the barriers which possible sexual embarrassment may cause.

We also need to look at men and their position in society. According to Forrester (1986), the traditional male sex stereotype is healthy, strong, independent and dominating. This hidden expectation can set barriers for men in seeking information about health education or preventive

Further information

For further educational material on TSE contact:

1. Yorkshire Regional Cancer Organisation
   Cookridge Hospital
   Leeds LS16 6QB

For a video demonstrating TSE, price £7.50 per copy.

2. Leaflets on TSE can be ordered free (up to 250 copies) from:
   Mr Evan Urquhart
   Senior Project Manager
   McCormack Ltd
   Church House
   Church Square
   Leighton Buzzard LU7 7AE.

Spread the message

References

Blesch, K.S. (1986) Health beliefs about testicular cancer and self-examination among professional men. *Oncology Nursing Forum,* **13,** 1, 29-33.

Carlin, P.J. (1986) Testicular self-examination: A public awareness program. *Public Health Reports,* **101,** 1, 98-102.

Conklin, M. et al (1978) Should health teaching include self-examination of the testis? *American Journal of Nursing,* **78,** 12, 2073-4.

Davies, J.M. (1981) Testicular cancer in England and Wales. *The Lancet,* **1,** 928-32.

Forrester, D.A. (1986) Myths of masculinity: Impact upon men's health. *Nursing Clinic North America,* **21,** 15-23.

Ganang, L.H. et al (1987) Young men's knowledge of testicular cancer and behavioural intentions towards testicular self-examination. *Patient Education Counselling,* **9,** 3, 251-61.

Thornhill, J.S. et al (1986) Public awareness of testicular cancer and the value of self-examination. *British Medical Journal,* **293,** 480-1.

health care. It can also prevent them from obtaining prompt medical advice for anything abnormal they might have detected, especially in areas affecting their sexuality. More health authorities should therefore be encouraged to set up 'Well Man' clinics, where men can obtain expert advice and receive regular check-ups. Men are also restricted in the time they can attend such services by their professional lives, and this should be taken into account by arranging evening or Saturday opening hours for such centres.

Finally, nurses must assess how the health education message could be spread among young and mostly healthy men, who rarely come into contact with their local hospital or consult their GP. On school entry, boys should be checked for undescended testicles and their parents need to be made aware of the associated risks. While in secondary school, boys could be introduced to TSE in sex education classes. This knowledge could later on be reinforced in colleges and universities during health care lectures or by promoting preventive medicine with the introduction of a 'self-care day'. Information boards with regularly changing topics on health and wellbeing could also be set up in the main meeting areas.

Male genitalia are particularly at risk of injury during sport exercises. PE teachers or sports trainers could therefore include information about TSE into their classes (Conklin et al, 1978).

During health screening in factories and companies, occupational nurses could assess the men's knowledge about testicular cancer and could encourage self-examination. Leaflets with detailed information should be available to bridge the possible embarrassment on both sides. The handout may be photocopied for this purpose and freely distributed to patients and clients.

As women are educated about breast examination, they should also be encouraged to inform their partners, husbands or brothers about TSE. It could also be taught to prospective fathers attending antenatal classes for lessons in parenting skills.

It is interesting to note that recent research has showed that the majority of men questioned had heard about TSE through the mass media and various instructional material; none of them had heard it from a nurse (Blesch, 1986). Information about TSE can be therefore very successfully spread through television or radio programmes and articles could be presented to local newspapers and magazines. Leaflets should be also made available in waiting rooms of hospitals, GPs' surgeries, health centres and public places like libraries. A small pamphlet on TSE could be included into condom packs.

Many recent health campaigns have focused around the early detection of women's diseases (eg, breast and cervical cancer). Men must also be involved in their own health screening and made aware that they are not immune from disease. Committed education programmes to inform men about testicular cancer and efficacy of TSE could save many lives at the moment being needlessly lost.

Testicular Self-Examination

As we are all responsible for our own health and wellbeing, we need to learn how to care for our own bodies and how to detect early abnormalities. Testicular cancer is a relatively rare disease, mainly affecting men between the age of 15 and 40 years. If the cancer is diagnosed and treated at an early stage, the cure rate is almost 100 per cent. Yet, if diagnosis is delayed it can be a fatal illness.

Monthly testicular examination is a simple procedure you yourself can do. If you find anything abnormal it isn't necessarily cancerous – there are many other conditions affecting the testicles – but it is important that you consult your doctor.

How to examine your testicles

1. Examine yourself on the first day of each month so you remember easily.
2. Following a warm bath or shower (the scrotum is then 'relaxed' and easier to examine) look at your scrotum in front of a mirror. The left side of the scrotum usually hangs lower than the right.
3. Feel the weight and size of each testicle.
4. Roll each testicle gently between your thumb and fingers (Figure 1).

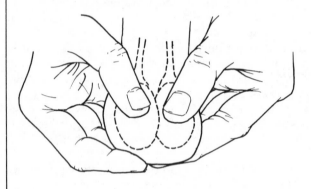

Figure 1. Roll each testicle gently between finger and thumb.

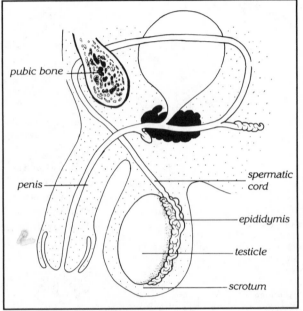

Figure 2. The spermatic cord extends up from the epididymis.

5. Locate the epididymis, which is a cord-like structure at the back of your testicle. It is always slightly tender when pressed. The spermatic cord extends upwards from the epididymis (Figure 2).
6. It will take a while to become confident in doing this self-examination.

CONTACT YOUR DOCTOR:

- If you can only feel one testicle in your scrotum (men with undescended testicles are at slightly greater risk of getting testicular cancer).

- If your scrotum is slightly enlarged and you have a feeling of dragging and heaviness. (Pain is experienced by very few patients.)

- If you have noticed a small lump or irregularity on the testicle.

- If you are simply unsure about how to examine yourself.

Remember:
If you notice anything unusual, it isn't necessarily cancerous. But don't delay in consulting your doctor; only he can make the final diagnosis.

Further information

For more information on testicular cancer, contact:
1. BACUP,
   121/123 Charterhouse Street,
   London EC1M 6AA.
   (Tel: 01-608 1661)
2. SOS (Save Our Sons),
   Shirley Wilcose, 1 Rite Hill, Wootton Bridge,
   Isle of Wight PO33 4LA.
3. Yorkshire Regional Cancer Organisation,
   Cookridge Hospital, Leeds LS16 6QB.

The Health Education Authority's recently launched campaign 'Look After Your Heart' has focused national attention on coronary heart disease, its causes, epidemiology and, most importantly on the personal strategies which individuals can adopt in order to minimise their own risk of developing CHD.

Preventing coronary heart disease

William Deans, RGN, RSCH, NV
Nurse Tutor, Wairiki College of Nursing, Rotarua, New Zealand

Robert Hoskins, RGN, RMN, NV
Development Officer with the Good Hearted Glasgow Campaign, Greater Glasgow Health Authority

A complex message

Providing clients with information about coronary heart disease (CHD) and its prevention, and with the incentive to use this information to change their own lifestyles is a massive task. The causes are numerous and complex, and medical controversy still rages over our understanding of the precise degree of importance of each of the causative factors. Changing peoples' attitudes and supporting them in changing their lifestyles is a difficult task, and the complexity of this particular health message compounds the challenge.

One essential component of all health education activities is that the individual's responsibility for his or her own health needs to be established. There is a widespread attitude among the general public that if the body goes wrong, it, and responsibility for it, can be 'handed over' to the health care professionals, to be fixed and mended. This is accompanied by the attitude that the individual has no real control, power or responsibility over the body's state of repair and disrepair in the first place. There is evidence that the climate of opinion of the general public is shifting a little on this issue (Health Education Authority, 1987), and the nursing profession has a strategic role in providing access to appropriately presented information and in supporting their clients in its use.

How to use the Heart Chart

The Heart Chart, which forms the handout overleaf, was designed to put the fun back into health, and to go some way towards encouraging individuals to take active responsibility for their own health, and to provide clients with at least some of the complex information relevant to the prevention of CHD (Deans and Hoskins, 1986). The chart can take the form of a contract, so that the patient is further encouraged to commit himself to try to make the changes in his lifestyle which he agrees are necessary. The technique of contracting involves the client's assumption of responsibility, and the idea of competing with oneself (to improve the score next time) actively puts the responsibility into the hands of the individual concerned.

Health Visitors, occupational health nurses and practice nurses are particularly well-placed to encourage clients to use the heart chart. Clients will need to agree to attend for regular screening checks, so that an individual health profile can be drawn up and subsequently reassessed. Details of family history of CHD, blood pressure, lung function, level of smoking, diet, weight, alcohol consumption, stress level and fitness should be assessed, and marked on the chart, by circling the appropriate recording against each heading.

The 'scores' in the top line can then be used to calculate a total score, which is compared with the three bands of the traffic signal at the top of the chart. Low scores give an indication of a reasonably low-risk lifestyle: roughly, the higher the score, the greater the risk. The heart

References
Deans, W. and Hoskins, R. (1986) — 'The Pilot Study of a New Community Service for Men.' Greater Glasgow Health Board.
Health Education Authority (1987): Attitudes to heart disease. HEA, London.

chart is not a scientific measure of risk, but does highlight the risk factors in an individual's present lifestyle, and can form the basis for the nurse to provide the client with the specific information required on the particular topics (such as smoking or diet).

One or two realistic, achievable goals for change can be agreed with the client, and recorded in the box on the top right hand corner of the chart, which they take away and keep. A time schedule for change could also be agreed, and a date booked for re-assessment health checks. The chart can be photocopied or adapted for use with patients and clients.

HEART CHART

21-40

DANGER
Your lifestyle needs
a major **overhaul**

11-20

CAUTION
There are several **blackspots**
requiring servicing

0-10

PROCEED
With care —
there may be **hazards** ahead

Your score is ☐

AREAS TO CHANGE
....
....
....

FAMILY HISTORY of high blood pressure or heart disease	None known	Possible but unsure	Extended family, eg cousins	Immediate family one relative	Immediate family 2 or more relatives
BLOOD PRESSURE diastolic	Normal	85-90	91-95	96-100	Over 100
LUNG EXPANSION Up to 100 Litres/min (men) and 85 l/m (women) below ideal score is within normal range	(Men) ideal (Women) ideal	50-74 45-64 below ideal score	75-99 65-84 below ideal score	100-149 85-134 below ideal score	150 or more 135 or more below ideal score
SMOKING Cigarettes per day	Non Smoker	Less than 5	5-9	10-19	More than 20
FAT IN DIET	No fried food Always use low fat foods	Fried foods once a week, low fat foods most days	Fried food twice a week, low fat food once a week	Fried food most days, low fat food occasionally	Fried food every day, never use low fat food
WEIGHT	Normal	½-1st overweight	1-1½st overweight	1½-2st overweight	2st or more overweight
ALCOHOL (Units per week) One unit = ½pt Beer/lager or one spirit, wine etc	(Men) 0-9 (Women) 0-4	10-19 5-9	20-35 10-19	36-49 20-27	50 or more 28 or more
STRESS	No more than usual	Occasional stress at home or work	Occasional stress at home and work	Considerable stress at home or work	Showing symptoms/on medication for stress
EXERCISE	3 times or more a week	Twice a week	Once a week	Once every 2-4 weeks	Less than once a month
AEROBIC FITNESS Step test	Excellent	Good	Average	Below average	Unable to complete

Adapted with kind permission from the Heart Chart devised by William Deans and Robert Hoskins

Although the principles involved in weight loss are straight-forward enough – less food, more exercise – many people have problems keeping to them. Crash diets, liquid diets are simply not the answer for realistic, long-term weight loss . . .

Not another diet?

Myra Ibbotson, PhD, BSc, SRD
Freelance Dietitian

Example: A woman who is 1.6m tall and weighs 60kg.

$$\frac{W}{H^2} = \frac{60}{1.6 \times 1.6}$$
$$= \frac{60}{2.56}$$
$$= 23.4$$

Her weight is therefore within the acceptable range.

Table 1. How to calculate body mass.

If you took a straw poll of friends and colleagues today, the chances are that a third would say they were 'slimming'. This preoccupation with weight is reflected on pharmacy shelves and in the classified pages of magazines: pills, machines, granules, teas and clothing are all available. Amidst all the hype it is easy to forget that the principles involved in losing weight are very simple. Energy expenditure should exceed energy intake for weight loss to occur. This can be achieved either by increasing expenditure (by taking more exercise) or by decreasing intake. Although the theory is simple, people find it very difficult to put into practice.

What is 'overweight'?

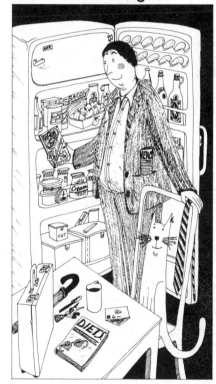

The body mass index or 'quetelet index' is the most reliable objective measure of overweight. It is calculated as weight/height^2 (in kg/m^2) (Table 1). This gives a single figure, thus avoiding the use of weight tables, which need to be interpreted with care. A body mass index of between 20 and 25 is acceptable: obesity is taken to start at 30, and gross obesity at 40.

In the vast majority of cases, obesity is primary – there is no predisposing condition. However, obesity does not necessarily mean gluttony. People have widely differing energy requirements, and in many cases a fat person actually eats less than a slim person. Many hypotheses for obesity have been proposed (such as a low basal metabolic rate, lack of brown adipose tissue or faulty appetite regulation), but none have been confirmed.

In a small number of obese people, an underlying mechanism such as an endocrinological disturbance can be found. Obesity can also follow a sudden drop in activity levels, such as bed rest following injury or arthritis. People can overeat for psychological reasons, too – food can be a solace when everything else seems to be going wrong, and, taken to extremes, this can obviously lead to weight gain.

The medical complications resulting from obesity increase both morbidity and mortality from a number of disorders, including coronary heart disease, respiratory disease, gallstones, diabetes and hypertension. Ironically, this is not as important for many people as the social pressure: exclusion from activities, the inability to wear fashionable clothes and the prejudice from a society in which overweight is unacceptable are probably more potent motivators than the threats to health.

Management of overweight

The most important role of the health professional in helping people to lose weight is to provide positive support and encouragement. Dieting is hard work: it means hunger and a constant battle of wills for most people. Any goals set must therefore be achievable and it is senseless to tell a woman who currently weighs 20 stones that she should aim for nine stones in as many months. A better approach is to tackle her weight loss in stages, for example, a stone at a time. Morale in people who have been overweight for a long time may be very low, and they may not have much confidence in their own ability to solve their problems.

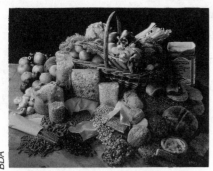

A sensible, well-balanced diet is more effective than crash diets.

Most people gain weight over a period of years rather than weeks, and the most effective long-term solution is to change eating and exercise patterns for life. The desire for an instant result is understandable, but the most common eventual outcome of short-term dieting is a return to old eating habits and a gradual regaining of all the weight lost so agonisingly while 'on the diet'. In addition, repeated short bursts on low calorie diets may lead to a lowering of the basal metabolic rate, so less energy can be consumed in order to maintain weight.

For this reason, crash diets or very low calorie liquid diets should not be advised. In the long term, they do not work and may endanger health in some cases. The points to be emphasised to the patient are:

- Long-term change is more important than short-term 'diets'. This means getting into the habit of buying lean meat, poultry or fish; eating plenty of fruit and vegetables; using wholegrain cereal products and low fat dairy products, and buying low-calorie versions of products such as soft drinks or salad dressings. Try to avoid buying foods such as biscuits that are especially tempting and nutritionally unimportant. Special diet foods such as meal replacement bars or drinks are unnecessary. Eat a variety of different foods each day.
- Have three regular meals a day. This helps to avoid hunger and the ensuing 'binge'.
- Try to cut intake by about a half, replacing foods especially high in fat or sugar with those listed above. (More details below.)
- Try to avoid alcohol.
- Aim for a realistic weight loss of between 0.5 to 1 kg per week.
- Some patients may find a group approach helpful. A good local slimming club (such as those run by *Slimming* magazine) could be recommended.
- If overeating is caused by emotional or psychological reasons, a dietary approach may be inappropriate: by imposing more stress on the patient it may even make the problem worse. Referral to a local group specialising in this type of eating disorder may be helpful. The patient may feel able to cope with a restrictive regimen once she stops seeing food as an emotional buffer.
- Keep a food diary, detailing everything eaten, where it was eaten, and mood at the time. This may reveal the amount of 'snacking' that is done unwittingly.

Drug therapy　The anorectic drugs available are used as an adjunct to diet therapy. They are most useful for patients with moderate to gross obesity, some of whom find themselves unbearably hungry on a reduced food intake. They do, however, have side-effects such as insomnia, raised blood pressure, irritability or psychotic reactions. For this reason their use cannot be justified in mild obesity.

Exercise　The benefits of exercise in a weight reduction regime are currently the focus of much attention. It is thought that exercise increases the resting metabolic rate even after it has finished, and that it decreases rather than increases appetite. In addition, an overweight person uses more energy than a thin person in doing the same exercise, because they have a heavier body to move.

How to Lose Weight

You may have decided to lose weight for a variety of reasons, such as a desire to look better or feel fitter. Your body will certainly be healthier as a result, because being overweight can predispose you to several medical conditions, such as heart disease, high blood pressure, diabetes, gallstones and arthritis. Unfortunately, there is no magic cure or diet; the only way to lose weight is by eating less food than your body needs. Don't do this by skipping meals or by following crash diets. Crash diets lead ultimately to weight gain. The guidelines which follow should help to ensure that loss is permanent by changing your food habits longterm.

Improve your eating behaviour

- Keep a food diary. Write down everything you eat or drink, whether you were hungry or not when you ate it and your mood at the time. This can be a real eye-opener to snacks consumed without noticing and times when you are vulnerable.
- Have three regular meals a day. Choose as wide a variety of foods as possible. Include foods from all of the food groups, ie, lean meat, fish or poultry, wholegrain cereals and bread, fruits and vegetables and low-fat dairy products every day.
- Eat in the same place, preferably sitting at a table. Do not read a paper or watch television while you are eating. Enjoy your food and eat slowly.
- Be tough over leftovers. Parents at home with small children may find they need to be extremely vigilant about throwing scraps away.
- Build some non-food rewards into your plan. This can be a visit to the hairdresser, a special outing, a book you've been longing to read . . . Whatever you do, though, don't buy clothes too small with a view to dieting into them.
- If you feel it would help to count calories, buy a reputable calorie counter (such as that produced by *Slimming* magazine). As a rough guide, women should aim for between 1,000 and 1,200kcal per day, and men 1,500 to 1,800kcal/day.
- Join a slimming club if you need moral support. *Slimming* magazine and Weightwatchers have clubs all over the country.
- If you want individual advice, ask your GP to refer you to your local dietetic department.

Shopping strategies

- Don't shop when you are hungry.
- Shop from a list and plan meals in advance.
- Don't buy foods which you find especially tempting. If you must buy them for a special treat, buy individual portions rather than family packs.

Increase your fibre intake

The main dietary principles are: *increase* your fibre intake and *decrease* your fat, sugar and alcohol intake. These are the same as current guidelines for healthy eating, and should form part of your long-term eating pattern.

- Use wholemeal bread.
- Eat plenty of fruit and vegetables of all varieties.
- Eat pulse vegetables (peas, beans and lentils).

They can be included in stews and casseroles.
- Use wholegrain cereals such as Weetabix, Shredded Wheat, Allbran or wheat flakes.
- Use brown rice or wholemeal pasta.

Decrease your fat and sugar intake

- Use a low fat spread (eg, Gold, Delight, Outline or supermarket own brands) instead of butter or margarine. (Note: margarines which are low in cholesterol or high in polyunsaturates contain the same calories as butter.)
- Use a low-fat milk (skimmed or semi-skimmed) instead of full fat (silver, red or gold top).
- Do not fry food. Get into the habit of grilling, poaching, stewing or steaming instead.
- Do not buy fatty meats such as breast of lamb or fatty meat products such as meat pies or pasties, salami and patés.
- Avoid fatty snacks such as crisps or nuts.

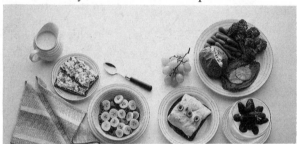

A nutritionally balanced daily slimming menu (From Slimming *Magazine's* Slimming Recipe Book*).*

- Buy lower fat versions of foods such as cheese and salad dressings.
- Do not use sugar in drinks. Instead use an artificial sweetener such as aspartame or Acesulfame k. Try different varieties of these until you find one that you like. They can also be used on cereals and in cooking (eg, stewing fruit).
- Do not buy sweets, chocolates or biscuits. If you are hungry between meals, have a piece of fruit.
- Use diet or slimline versions of soft drinks. Many taste the same as the real thing. Or try a fizzy mineral water with ice and lemon.
- Avoid sweet puddings. Instead have some fruit or a low fat/low sugar yoghurt.
- Avoid alcohol. High in calories, it is also an appetite stimulant, so you'll probably eat more.

High days and holidays

- On special occasions, relax your diet and enjoy yourself.
- Make allowance for a bigger meal in the evening by cutting down earlier in the day.
- If you do break your diet, don't despair. Just start again the next day.

Useful reading

DHSS (1987) COMA report, no. 31, The use of very low calorie diets in obesity. HMSO, London.

Garrow, J.S. (1981) Treat Obesity Seriously. Churchill Livingstone, Edinburgh.

Orbach, S. (1984) Fat is a Feminist Issue. Hamlyn, London.

Truswell, A.S. (1986) Obesity: Diagnosis and risks: causes and management. In: ABC of Nutrition. British Medical Association, London.

Since their first appearance in 1887, contact lenses have been developed immeasurably, and now are used to treat many conditions.

Part of your daily routine: teaching good contact lens care

Julie T. Cotgreave, RGN; ONC; Tracy M. Patch, RGN; Carolyne E. Perthen, RGN, RSCN; Avril B. Stewart, RGN, RSCN; Kathleen Crutchlow, RGN

This paper was written while the authors were students on the Ophthalmic Nursing course at Coventry and Warwickshire Hospital and Paybody Eye Hospital Coventry

The first suggestion that a lens coming into contact with the eye could be used to correct vision came from Leonardo da Vinci, back in 1508, but it was not until 1827 that a practical method of making a lens was suggested by Sir John Herschel. The first lenses known to be fitted were made by a German optician, F. E. Mueller in 1887. They were extremely large glass 'haptic lenses' that covered the entire eye and could usually only be worn for about two hours at a time.

The great advances in contact lens manufacturing came with the introduction of plastics. Initially, British manufacturers used the new plastics to make haptic lenses and later developed 'micro lenses' which were smaller than the cornea. Today there are a number of different types of lens:
- hard perspex;
- gas permeable;
- soft;
- bifocal;
- tinted.

Optical and medical uses

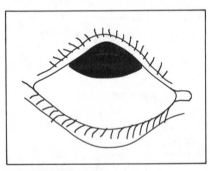

Figure 1. Keratoconus.

Contact lenses can be used for medical and optical reasons. The medical reasons for wearing a contact lens make constant visits to the hospital necessary to adjust its fittings. A lens can be placed in front of the eye to improve visual acuity or appearance in various circumstances. The most common are described here.

Keratoconus This condition is thought to be hereditary, but it is more common in men and associated with people who suffer from chronic allergies. The cornea becomes conical in shape (Figure 1), but once the contact lens is fitted the uneven surface of the cornea is rendered smooth so that light entering the eye focuses more clearly on the macula. Another similar condition is keratoconus posticus, in which the cornea bulges backward (the opposite effect of keratoconus), but this cannot be corrected by a contact lens.

Corneal grafts (keratoplasty) The cornea of a donor's eye is transplanted into the eye of a recipient. Over 60 per cent of transplants are successful, and a few surgeons use a contact lens postoperatively to support the transplanted tissue. As the newly operated eye is very sensitive, close monitoring is important. Using a contact lens in this way may help to reduce astigmatism.

Raised corneal scars Corneal scars normally occur when an external object pierces the cornea. When the tissue begins to heal, scar tissue is formed, and a haptic lens can be used to smooth and reduce the proudness of the scar.

Cosmetic A haptic lens can improve the appearance of an eye, by occluding any abnormalities such as aniridia or iris holes.

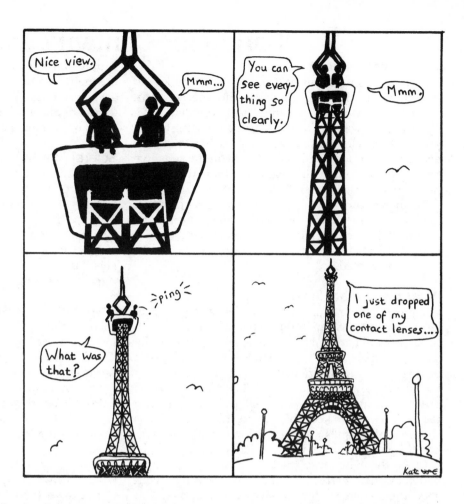

The handout overleaf can be photocopied and given to patients and clients.

Acknowledgements
We would like to thank the following people for their help and encouragement while we were preparing this project: Dr. H. Farrell, Principal Optician, Coventry and Warwickshire Hospital, Coventry. Mr. I. Stewart, Husband of Mrs. A. Stewart, for his illustrations. Miss J. McCrae, Sister, Outpatients Department, Coventry and Warwickshire Hospital, Coventry. Mrs. S.M. Parr, Tutor, Coventry Ophthalmic Nurse Training School.

References
Ruben, M. (1975) Contact Lens Practice.Balleire Tindall.
Stollery, R. (1987) Ophthalmic Nursing. Blackwell Scientific, Oxford.

Extended wear and bandage lenses

Bullous keratopathy   In this condition the cornea becomes 'water-logged' (oedematous). This causes pain, epiphora (lacrimmation), photophobia and diplopia. By inserting a soft contact lens, compression is applied which helps to reduce corneal oedema.

Symblepharon   In this condition, the palpebral and bulbar conjunctiva are adherent. It is caused by burns or inflammation. The lens helps to prevent these adhesions.

Exposure keratitis   Retraction of the eyelids is caused by damage to the seventh cranial nerve. The corneal surface is exposed and dries out, and the normally clear cornea becomes cloudy. To prevent this, a soft lens may be employed to preserve the tear film (Ruben, 1975).

Drug administration   A soft contact lens may be impregnated with a drug which is then slowly released, usually over 12 hours (Stollery, 1987).

Albinism   This is a condition in which there is an absence of pigmentation, giving the typical appearance of white hair, pale skin and pink eyes. Cosmetic improvement can be achieved by using tinted soft lenses (Ruben, 1975).

Aphakia   The lens of the eye is removed by surgery, leaving the eye without one of its focusing curvatures. Soft or hard contact lenses can be used to realign the light entering the eye (Stollery, 1987).

Refractive errors   Most errors of refraction such as myopia, hypermetropia and astigmatism (a condition in which the cornea does not focus light evenly due to irregular curvatures) can be easily corrected by contact lenses (Stollery, 1987).

First introduced in America, these are essentially similar to soft lenses but have a higher water content. They are softer and allow more oxygen to reach the cornea, so they can be worn for up to three months. Consequently they are suitable for babies, elderly and handicapped people to use.

Caring for Contact Lenses

Getting your lenses

To obtain contact lenses you have to make an appointment with your optician who specialises in assessing people's eyesight. A complete eye examination will be carried out to determine the prescription of lenses you need, and the health of your eyes and your body. Additional tests on the sensitive tissues at the front of your eyes determine which lens material may be successfully used for you.

Taking account of your visual needs, environment, special activities and personal preferences, the optician will decide which lens to recommend to you. Not everybody can wear the same type of lens, so you have to be guided.

What are contact lenses?

The most common type of contact lenses are corneal lenses, which are small, thin, shell-like discs that fit onto the front curvature of the eye, and are practically invisible when worn. They are made from high grade optical plastic. Moisture that is constantly present on the surface of your eye provides a cushion on which the lenses can float. As they are light in weight, they require no more to keep them in position than what is known as the capillary attraction of the moisture layer and the gentle touch of the eyelids.

When the eye moves, the lens moves too, giving a better visual correction than is possible with spectacles. There are three main reasons for this:

- There is no restriction in your visual field when looking straight ahead.
- When you turn your eye, the lens moves with it so all the images you see pass through the lens. You cannot look past the edge of the lens, as you can with spectacles.
- Objects all appear a more natural size, whatever your eye prescription, than they do with spectacles.
  There are four main types of contact lenses.

Hard lenses

Hard lenses are very small (about 9mm in diameter) and are produced from rigid plastic. They provide excellent vision and are generally less expensive than other types of contact lenses. The care routine to look after them is very easy to follow and quickly becomes part of your normal way of life.

Soft lenses

Soft lenses are made from a flexible water absorbent material which allows oxygen, which is required by the eye, to pass through the lens. They may require replacement more frequently than other types of lens and require particular attention to cleaning and care routines. Soft lenses can be worn periodically if required, but are usually used for daily wear.

Gas permeable

Gas permeable lenses are a comparatively new development and are made from a plastic which has been developed specifically to combine many of the advantages of hard and soft lenses. The eye requires a supply of oxygen to maintain it in a healthy state, and the main advantage of these lenses is that they allow oxygen to pass through to the eye. The care systems for gas permeable lenses are straightforward and they offer an excellent standard of vision.

Scleral (haptic) lenses

Scleral lenses fit over the cornea and sclera (the outer coating of the eyeball), although only the corneal section of the lens corrects visual defects. These lenses, although bulky, cannot fall out and are easier for poorly sighted people to handle. They are used mainly for the diseased eye and need specialist fitting. They are also used for people who take part in vigorous sporting activities.

Preparation for wearing lenses

Follow a routine.

1. Wash your hands with a mild soap, to reduce the risk of introducing infection into the eye.
2. Rinse hands and dry them with a lint free towel (one that does not shed fibres).
3. Start with the right lens first, removing it from compartment marked (R).
4. Inspect the lens to see if it is clean, wet and not torn.

Points to remember

1. Always wash your hands and dry them on a lint free towel before touching your lenses.
2. Cleaning and disinfecting your lenses is important to prevent eye infections. Do it every day.
3. Take care not to tear soft lenses. Keep your nails short.
4. Start your routine with the same lens each time to avoid mixing right and left.
5. Don't clean your lens over a sink with the plug out.
6. If you have any problems, consult your practitioner.
7. Corneal and conjunctival irritation may occur if you handle your lenses after chopping chillies. This is caused by the chilli fluid lingering on your hands and contaminating the lenses on removal.

Caring for your lenses

It is essential that you establish a regular and thorough care routine for your lenses. If you do not, you may get serious disorders of the eye. Daily care for soft and gas permeable lenses consists of cleaning, rinsing and disinfecting with recommended solutions. Remove, clean, rinse and disinfect extended wear lenses once weekly.

Proteins build up on the surfaces of soft and gas permeable. Remove the build up of these proteins once every week on soft lenses, and once a fortnight on gas permeable lenses. Hard lenses do cause some drying of the cornea and may be uncomfortable to wear. To overcome this a wetting solution should be used.

continued . . .

Inserting your lenses

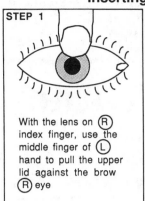

STEP 1

With the lens on Ⓡ index finger, use the middle finger of Ⓛ hand to pull the upper lid against the brow Ⓡ eye

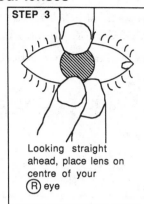

STEP 3

Looking straight ahead, place lens on centre of your Ⓡ eye

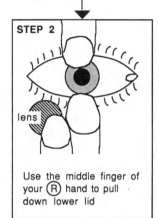

STEP 2

lens

Use the middle finger of your Ⓡ hand to pull down lower lid

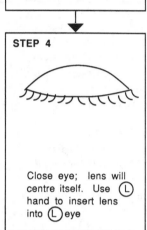

STEP 4

Close eye; lens will centre itself. Use Ⓛ hand to insert lens into Ⓛ eye

Your questions answered

Q. Can anyone wear contact lenses?

A. Yes, with advice from an optician.

Q. Do other people notice them?

A. Very rarely.

Q. Are they comfortable?

A. There is some discomfort at first, particularly with hard lenses. You must follow the wearing schedule as advised by your optician. It is important not to exceed your recommended wearing time – overwearing can cause discomfort.

Q. What are the advantages of contact lenses?

A. The main reasons people wear contact lenses are cosmetic. They find them more acceptable than spectacles. Also, specially tinted lenses can be made to conceal unsightly marks and squints. There are practical reasons for choosing them too:
- They give a larger field of unobstructed vision.
- They do not steam up with changes in temperature.
- The rain presents no problem to wearers.

Q. Can I wear eye make-up with contact lenses?

A. Yes, but insert your lenses first.

Q. Should I use special eye make-up?

A. Liquid eye shadow is preferable, and powder eyeliners that can be mixed with water are recommended. It is best to use cheaper mascara, as it is dissolvable and can be removed completely.

Q. Do I need to take care when applying face creams?

A. Yes, apply all creams *after* inserting your lenses.

Q. Can I use hairspray?

A. Yes, providing you shield your eyes.

Q. Can I have my hair permed or coloured?

A. Fumes from permanent waves are very irritating to

lens wearers. Permanent tints and dyes are safer than hair rinses which contain metal particles which cause corneal abrasions. One final word about hair care – it is inadvisable to sit under a hair dryer, as the hot air dries both the tear film and the plastic of the lens, causing it to rub on the eye.

Q. Can I play sports while wearing contact lenses?

A. Yes, soft or haptic lenses are advised, as the other types are easily dislodged. It is not advisable to swim while wearing any contact lenses.

Q. Do I need a pair of spectacles?

A. Yes, for use in emergencies.

Q. Can I wear ordinary sun glasses?

A. Yes. Contact lens wearers have much more freedom of choice.

Q. Can the lens slip around the back of the eye?

A. No.

Q. Can I sleep in contact lenses?

A. No, unless they are extended wear lenses.

Q. Should I insure my lenses?

A. Yes, your optician will normally arrange this.

Removing your lenses

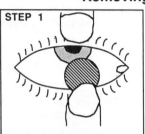

STEP 1

Look up slowly. Pull down lower lid with middle finger of Ⓡ hand. With Ⓡ index finger slide lens down to lower white of eye

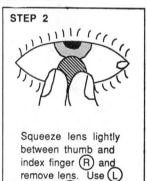

STEP 2

Squeeze lens lightly between thumb and index finger Ⓡ and remove lens. Use Ⓛ hand for Ⓛ eye.

If a lens is uncomfortable

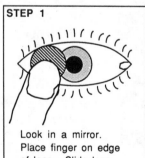

STEP 1

Look in a mirror. Place finger on edge of lens. Slide lens away from nose, while looking towards your nose

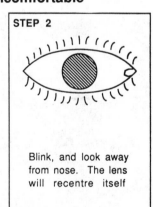

STEP 2

Blink, and look away from nose. The lens will recentre itself

We hope this handout has given you a better insight into contact lenses, and helped you to decide whether or not you would like to wear them. Your optician will be only too willing to take time to explain the care that is required. It is essential to keep meticulous hygiene standards when looking after your lenses.

Remember, you only have one pair of eyes – look after them!

As the incidence of AIDS and HIV infection rises, nurses have an increasing role in caring for sufferers. They are also in a position to educate the public abouit the virus.

Professional care for people with HIV/AIDS

James Stanford, BA, RGN, NDN
District Nurse, Brighton Community Nursing Service

AIDS is increasing in incidence and as yet there is no certain medical cure for the syndrome. Health education is the only 'vaccine' currently available. Well informed nurses who have a positive attitude are in a position to give both high quality nursing care and sound educational advice. Health education is usually most effective when given on a one to one basis, and nurses are often in such a privileged position, and are therefore able to give direct and effective advice to their patients. The handout on page 85 provides up-to-date information about AIDS and the HIV virus; it can be photocopied for distribution to patients and clients.

AIDS is a disease in which impaired immunity results in serious secondary infection and tumours. It can also directly affect the central nervous system. The primary cause of the disease is a virus known as human immunodeficiency virus, (HIV). Acquiring the virus *may* result in developing clinical AIDS after a variable incubation period, although most people who are HIV antibody positive have not yet developed AIDS.

Transmission of the virus

The virus can be transmitted in three ways: blood, blood products or donated organs; via sexual intercourse and from mother to fetus.

Blood products   The virus is present in the blood even when the individual is symptomless, and all blood must be considered a hazard. Blood presents the main hazard to health care staff. Saliva, faeces, vomit and urine are not considered a hazard unless contaminated with blood, but it is not always obvious if blood is present, so caution needs to be taken when handling these fluids. The virus is readily destroyed by heat and suitable disinfectants. The use of unsterilised syringes and needles by iv drug users is the main source of transmission via blood in this country.

Sexual transmission   HIV can be present in semen, and sexual intercourse is the commonest mode of transmission. While it appears to occur more readily during anal intercourse, transmission can occur during vaginal intercourse. The use of condoms is essential in reducing the risk of such transmission. However, condoms can fail and complete safety cannot be assured.

Mother to child   The virus can be transmitted from mother to child before or during birth. A significant proportion of children born to mothers who are HIV antibody positive will themselves be antibody positive and may develop AIDS. Pregnancy can also increase the risk to an antibody positive woman of developing AIDS.

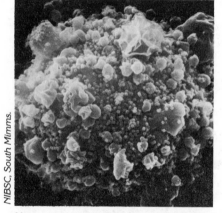

NIBSC, South Mimms.

Human immunodeficiency virus (the small spherical particles) budding from the surface of an infected T-lymphocyte (cultured cell); magnification x 20,000.

Nursing patients with HIV/AIDS

Open ward or side room   Most patients can be nursed on an open ward. A side room is only necessary if there is severe bleeding or diarrhoea or if their general condition indicates it.

Bibliography

Altman, D. (1986) AIDS and the New Puritanism. Pluto Press, London.
The political and social implications of HIV/AIDS.

Miller, D., Weber, J., Green, J. (Eds) (1986) The Management of AIDS Patients. Macmillan, London.
Medical information and practical nursing guidance.

Miller, D. (1987) Living with AIDS and HIV. Macmillan, London.
A practical book on medical and psychological aspects of HIV/AIDS.

Pratt, R.J. (1986) AIDS: A strategy for Nursing Care. Edward Arnold, London.
Written specifically for nurses.

RCN (1986) Nursing Guidelines on the Management of Patients in Hospital and the Community suffering from AIDS. Second Report of the RCN AIDS Working Party.

Shilts, R. (1987) And the band played on: Politics, People and the AIDS epidemic. Penguin group, London.
A journalistic view documenting the history of HIV/AIDS in America.

Tatchell, P. (1986) AIDS: A Guide to Survival. Heretic Books, GMP, London.
A good general read.

Plastic apron and gloves These should be used when giving direct patient care involving handling body fluids, and also when dealing with spillages or handling specimens.

Barrier nurse This is necessary when the patient has tuberculosis, salmonella or severe herpes.

Handwashing and hand care Before and after patient care procedures, scrupulous hand care should be observed. Cuts must be covered with waterproof plasters.

Disposal of needles Needles should not be resheathed, bent or broken, and should be disposed of in the sharps container by the patient's bed. There is no need to separate unless taking blood, then the needle should be removed from the syringe and disposed of, the specimen jar filled and the syringe put in the sharps container. All specimens should be placed in a bag marked with a biohazard label.

General disinfection In the event of blood spills, use undiluted hypochlorite solution (Melzone) or domestic bleach (domestos, parazone etc), leave for 10 minutes and mop up using paper towels and gloves.

Disinfection of equipment Disposable equipment is not specifically required. If contaminated by bood, nursing equipment can be disinfected using Melzone or bleach with paper towels and gloves.

Blood contaminated materials All blood contaminated rubbish should be disposed of in double bags marked 'for incineration'.

Crockery and cutlery There is no need for separate utensils unless the patient has a mouth infection.

Linen Linen, including soiled linen, can be washed in the normal way. If contaminated by blood, wash separately on hot wash cycle of the washing machine. If sent to the hospital laundry, linen contaminated by blood should be double bagged in dissolvable laundry bags.

Toilet facilities Ambulant patients do not need separate toilet or washing facilities. After use they can be cleaned in the normal manner and any spillages in the toilets disinfected with Melzone or bleach. Disposable nappies and inco sheets should be double bagged and disposed of in the usual way.

Reducing the spread

Nurses can do too much to help reduce the spread of HIV and AIDS.
- Learn about HIV/AIDS.
- Follow these guidelines on the prevention of infection.
- Inform the public about HIV/AIDS, and help dispel the myths and prejudices.
- Encourage everyone to accept responsibility for their sexual relationships and activities, and so protect themselves and their partners' health.
- Encourage the use of condoms.
- Encourage intravenous drug users not to share needles and syringes and to practise safer sex.
- Inform the public about donating blood. There is no risk to the donor. Allay anxieties about blood transfusions – the risk is negligible.
- Encourage people with HIV to adopt a healthy lifestyle, and tell them how to avoid infecting others.
- Know where to go for specialised help and counselling.
- Promote a caring and responsible attitude towards people who have the virus.

The handout overleaf can be photocopied and distributed to patients.

Reducing Your Risk from AIDS

AIDS (acquired immune deficiency syndrome) is a disease caused by the human immunodeficiency virus (HIV). This virus can destroy white blood cells, thereby impairing the body's defence systems, leaving the body vulnerable to infections, which can be serious or fatal. People with AIDS may develop particular, and often rare, forms of cancer or serious infections in the lungs, digestive system, and the central nervous system. Most people who have HIV do not have AIDS, and many are unlikely to develop it. However, the onset of AIDS after infection with HIV can be anything from 12 weeks to at least eight years and the long term outlook for people who have been infected with the virus is uncertain.

How is the virus passed on?

The three ways in which the virus can be transmitted are via blood, blood products or donated organs: through penetrative sex and from mother to fetus. The virus can exist in saliva and tears, but in such small quantities that it is not transmittable by normal contact with these fluids.

Blood

If you are a drug user who injects, always use your own syringes and needles. Never share with anyone, no matter how well they may appear. When you have finished with your needle, bend it back and put it in a tin which can be put in a dustbin or burnt. If you inject yourself using an unsterilised needle and syringe you could become infected with HIV if the equipment has been used by somebody with the virus.

● Avoid sharing any device that punctures the skin, unless it has been properly sterilised. This includes hypodermic needles, syringes, earpiercing equipment, tattooing and acupuncture needles. Any needles or syringes which doctors, nurses or dentists use more than once are always properly sterilised each time. There is no risk of getting infected by donating blood to the National Blood Transfusion Service, because a new needle is used for each donor. In Britain all blood and blood products are now screened to minimise the risk of infection from receiving a transfusion. Before this precaution was taken, there were a number of cases of infection, particularly of people with haemophilia.

● To prevent infected blood from entering your body, it's best not to share razors or toothbrushes. People often nick themselves when shaving, and many people's gums bleed when they brush their teeth.

Safer sex

The most common way the virus is transmitted is through sexual contact. HIV does not affect people because of who they are, but because of what they do. Any one can catch the disease, not just gay men – it is the sexual activities of the individual that create the risks. Each of us is responsible for our own health and wellbeing and must accept that responsibility by being aware of the principles of safer sex.

● Kissing and cuddling are safe. Masturbation, body rubbing and massage are also safe.

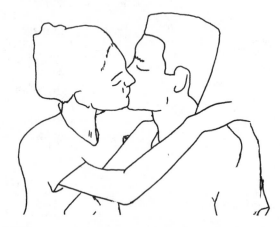

● Oral sex – sucking – is also safe, providing no semen enters your mouth. There is an element of risk if you allow semen to enter your mouth, because if you have cuts or sores in your mouth or gums, the virus could enter the blood stream.

● Vaginal intercourse is risky. Anal intercourse is even more risky, because of the delicate nature of the lining of the rectum, which is liable to sustain small breaks and tears. Using a condom during intercourse will reduce the risk of getting the virus. If you use a lubricant with the condom, make sure it is a water based one, such as KY. Oil-based ones, such as Vaseline, tend to weaken the rubber. You should always use a lubricant during anal intercourse, to reduce the possibility of the condom splitting. Condoms are not completely reliable, because they can fail. Intercourse, even with a condom, does carry some risk.

● Reducing your number of sexual partners will reduce the chance of you coming into contact with someone with the virus. However, this will only affect your chances of catching the virus if you have sex that involves an element of risk. You only need to do something risky (such as having intercourse without a condom) with one person who has the virus to catch it. On the other hand, you can do something completely safe (such as masturbation) with any number of people and run no risk of catching the virus.

Mothers

The virus can be transmitted from mother to child before or during birth. A significant proportion of children born to mothers who are HIV antibody positive will themselves be antibody positive and may develop AIDS. Pregnancy can also increase the risk to an antibody positive woman of developing AIDS. Mothers who are considered to be at high risk of having the HIV virus are offered counselling and a special blood test during their pregnancy.

If you know someone with HIV

Few illnesses have created such a climate of alarm, prejudice and moral panic; inevitably this has affected our attitudes towards people with HIV or AIDS who are often stigmatised as a result. Attitudes towards related issues, such as homosexuality, drug users, promiscuity, sexually transmitted diseases and death reinforce prejudice. We all need to think through our attitudes and to be aware of their effects on others. People with the virus can feel very isolated. You can help them by not treating them differently.

There is no possibility of catching the virus from ordinary day-to-day contact with someone who has the virus. There's no need to have separate cups, glasses, plates or cutlery. You can't catch AIDS from a toilet seat, from holding hands, from food or clothing.

The only care needed is with spilt blood. This should be cleaned up – if possible by the person it comes from. Put on rubber gloves and wipe up the blood with paper towels and bleach.

If there is a child with the HIV virus at your child's school, there is no danger of the virus being passed on during ordinary school activities. If you are at all worried, talk to your child's headteacher.

How to tell if you have HIV

There is a special blood test called the HIV antibody blood test. It shows whether you have developed antibodies to the virus. Whenever a new virus enters your bloodstream, your blood builds up antibodies to fight it off, after a period of two to eight weeks.

If the test shows that you have the antibodies, it means you have been in contact with the virus. But there is no test that will tell if you will go on to develop AIDS, or when this may happen.

If you think you might have the virus and you want to have the blood test, think about it carefully. The drawbacks may well outweigh the advantages. For example, you may find it very difficult to get life insurance or a mortgage once you have had the test, regardless of the result. Before having the test, it may help to talk to a health adviser, to work out how you would cope with the result if the test shows that you have been in contact with the virus.

If any doctor wants to take a blood specimen from you to test for HIV antibodies she or he should obtain your permission beforehand. Make sure you know what your doctor may be testing your blood for, and that your consent is sought.

You can get advice about having the test from any of the organisations listed below.

Staying healthy

The best bet is to heed the advice in this handout! If you already are antibody positive, it is still important to practise safer sex, both to protect your sexual partner/s and to protect yourself from further infections which may further compromise your immune system. Alchohol depresses the immune system and can increase the body's risk of acquiring infection. Stress also depresses the immune system and hence threatens anyone's health. Relaxation exercises and meditation are just two ways of coping with stress. A healthy balanced diet will also help you to stay healthy. There are various complementary therapies which many people find helpful. Further information can be obtained from The Institute of Complementary Medicine, telephone 01-636 9543.

Further Information

STD (sexually transmitted disease) clinics.
STD clinics give free, confidential advice and treatment. Look in the 'phone book for the number of your local clinic.

Terrence Higgins Trust
52–54 Grays Inn Road, London WC1X 8LT. Telephone helpline 01-833 2971 Daily 3pm-10pm. The Trust offers help and counselling to people with HIV virus or AIDS, and their friends and relatives. Detailed information on safer sex and advice on the HIV antibody test are available. They can also put you in touch with local AIDS helplines.

London Lesbian and Gay Switchboard
01-837 7234 (24hrs). The switchboard can answer general queries about HIV/AIDS, put you in touch with local gay support groups and local AIDS helplines.

National AIDS Helpline
0800 567 123. A 24 hour service. Calls are free, and the Helpline offers confidential information, advice and, where necessary, referral to appropriate counselling agencies. For the deaf and hard of hearing, on Minicom: 0800 521361 10am-10pm.

SCODA (Standing Conference on Drug abuse)
01-430 2341. SCODA has a full list of local services for drug users throughout the country.

Part of this handout has been adapted, with kind permission, from the Health Education Authority's booklet 'AIDS: what everybody needs to know'. This booklet is out of print, but a new up-to-date series of leaflets is available from your local health education unit, or from: Dept A, PO Box 100, Milton Keynes, MK1 1TX.

Babies and Children

Faecal incontinence in children requires not only treatment for the child but also support for the family. Many encopretic conditions can be exacerbated by the natural anxiety that parents feel about their child.

Encopresis: family support must accompany treatment

Arthur F. Turner, BA, RGN, DNCert
Community Liaison Officer, Newport, Gwent

For most parents the training of their child's bowels occurs between one and 2½ years of age. This is often initiated either due to family tradition or following advice from the family health visitor. By the age of four, 89 per cent of children will be totally in control (Largo and Stutyle, 1977). Despite this, constipation remains very common, and in certain circumstances encopresis can follow.

Much can be done to help encopretic children and their families by the primary health care team (or continence advisor). An individual care plan can be developed that supports the family as a unit, as many encopretic conditions can be exacerbated by ignorance and anxiety.

Influences prior to encopresis

Training for faecal continence is usually based on the gastrocolic reflex – the peristaltic wave that occurs after a meal that pushes faeces from the colon into the rectum, initiating the desire to defaecate. Many parents believe that sitting their young babies on a potty and thereby utilising these reflexes can potty train them. However, most children do not have the physical or mental maturity to be able to fully control their bowels until about 18 months old, so the potty training is for convenience only – although most people would agree that it is much better than cleaning a number of soiled nappies daily. Coupled to the potty training is an element of praise and encouragement which reinforces the child's approved behaviour (in this case passing its faeces in the potty) while the child becomes aware of the sensation associated with a full rectum.

There are many factors affecting the consistency of stools, and these can strongly influence the child's ability to become faecally continent. They include diet, amount drunk and exercise. If the stools are hard and consequently difficult to pass, the child may begin to associate the potty or toilet with pain and thereby learn a pattern of behaviour that contributes towards constipation and delayed learning of faecal continence. This delayed pattern of behaviour can also occur when there is a transition from the potty to the toilet. The child may feel much safer opening his or her bowels in the semi-squat position produced by sitting on the potty. The praise that normally went with the use of the potty is often abruptly halted, while the child is expected to open his or her bowels while teetering on an uncomfortable toilet.

The position adopted as a result is not ideal for the natural response of the body to close the epiglottis and lower the diaphragm in order to help the expelling of the faeces and assist the peristaltic contractions (valsalva's response). Children cannot produce much push if their feet are unsupported, so they need, as a basic requirement, a child's toilet seat, as well as somewhere to rest their legs.

Parental response

There is also a link between encopresis and the parents' response to soiled nappies when the child is very young. If the child only receives attention when he has soiled nappies and is otherwise unstimulated and

Bibliography

Jones, C. (1985) Encopresis. *American Journal of Nursing*, **85,** 154-156.
  A nursing article highlighting the fear-pain cycle.
Loening Baucka, V.A. and Cruikshank, B.M. (1986) Abnormal defaecation dynamics in chronically constipated children with encopresis. *The Journal of Paediatrics*, **108,** 4.
  A study highlighting the dangers of long-term constipation.
O'Regan et al (1986) Constipation – a commonly unrecognised cause of enuresis. *AJDC*, **140, 261-1.**
  An interesting article linking enuresis with constipation.
Perkins, M. et al (1985) Diagnosis and management of constipation and encopresis in childhood. *Texas Medicine*, **81.**
  A clear guide to enable an accurate diagnosis and sensible management programme.

References

Bellman, M. (1966) Studies of encopresis. *Acta Pediatr Scan*, **170**, 1, supplement.

Bennett, M. (1988) The fibre squad. *Nursing Times*, **84**, 4, 49.

Hussian, S.A. (1984) Childhood psychiatric disorders with physical manifestations. *Indian J. Pediat*, **51**, 205-216.

Landman, G.B. and Rappaport, L. (1985) Pediatric management of severe treatment resistant encopresis. *Dev. and Behav. Pediatrics*, **6**, 6, 349-51.

Largo, R.H. and Stutzle, W. (1977) Longitutional study of bowel and bladder control by day and at night in the first six years of life, I: epidemiology and interrelations between bowel and bladder control. *Developmental Child Neurology*, **19**, 598-606.

Levine, M.D. and Badkow, H. (1976) Children with encopresis: a study of treatment outcomes. *Pediatrics*, **58**, 845-852.

Lowry, S.P. et al (1985) Habit training as a treatment of encopresis secondary to chronic constipation. *Journal of Paediatric Gastroenterology and Nutrition*, **4**, 397-401.

Rolder, A. and van Houten, R. (1985) Treatment of constipation-caused encopresis by a negative reinforcement procedure. *Journal of Behav. and Exp. Psychiat*, **16**, 1, 67-70.

Continued on page 40

Encopresis

The three types of encopresis are roughly:
1. The child who has never been trained who may come from a deprived family whose lifestyle mitigates against formal training.
2. The child who may regress from continence after a period of faecal continence.
3. The child who has faecal incontinence/soiling due to retention and constipation.

Reducing stress

neglected, this can give rise, when the child is older, to a pattern of soiling, psychologically learnt from babyhood to gain attention from adults. Although a strict toilet training regime at too early an age is not recommended, if the child is not introduced to the potty or toilet in a relaxed fashion soon enough, he can become used to passing faeces in a nappy, often preferring to become constipated than use the receptacle his parents have belatedly offered. This can begin to create the stress in toiletting activities that is so common in the families of encopretic children.

Another important facet to faecal continence is the availability of the toilet. Many household routines do not allow time for opening of the bowels, especially in the rush of the morning and this 'refusing the call to stool' is often responsible for defective excretory patterns later on in childhood. The rectum of such children becomes stretched and desensitised and this leads to a chronic condition of the bowel, where the bowel becomes grossly distended by the backlog of faecal matter. This blockage prevents the normal cycle of elimination and a spurious diarrhoea presents as liquid faecal matter and leaks its way around the obstruction. Diet has a strong influence on the normal workings of the bowels, as food high in roughage assists in the passage of the forming stool and makes defaecation considerably easier. Although some families have been giving their children too much dietary fibre, children in the main are allowed to be too conservative in their selection of food. The appeal of fast, convenient foods lures them towards a diet high in fat and lacking in fibre. Meals like beefburgers and chips are so popular with children that it is not surprising constipation is a common problem, and the setting up of constipation clinics in some health authorities highlights this (Bennett, 1988).

Encopresis, or faecal incontinence, is not a very common complaint but it gives rise to much more repulsion and distress than enuresis. One study suggested that it affected about one per cent of five-year-olds (Bellman, 1966), but a later study put the figure as high as 1½ per cent of seven to eight year-olds (Schaefer, 1979). This is only a tenth of the incidence of enuresis. Many of the studies that have been conducted into encopresis have highlighted the role of stress in the appearance and continuation of faecal soiling and many of the effective treatments concentrate on ways of removing anxiety from the child's environment. Much of this work has been done in England and will be described later.

Investigators (eg, Hussain, 1984) have tried to categorise types of encopresis, and while these distinctions are not mutually exclusive they do appear to give some framework to the professional to enable a rational form of treatment to be carefully thought out and implemented.

By far the easiest way of reducing stress (and the cornerstone of most of the treatment options that have been described involves the reduction of stress) is to try to get the parents or carers to praise the behaviour that they wish for from the child and to remove from their interaction with the child any form of retribution associated with the soiling or faecal incontinence. Implementing this however, is fraught with problems. It may be perfectly natural to get aggressive and short-tempered with a child that soils but it is the primary way of reinforcing his/her negative behaviour; in contrast, praise is one of the most effective forms of discipline. A programme must be formulated in order for a logical approach to treatment to be written down and the staff and carers involved must have a good idea as to the direction of that treatment.

Encopresis is often secondary to chronic constipation and very often these cases are extremely resistant to treatment. Some of the problems may be caused by the ignorance of the parents or carers as to the exact function of the bowel. This requires the practitioner to have a good relationship with the family so that a 'demystification' process can be undertaken (Landman and Rappaport, 1985). This is vital, and considerable time needs to be spent on it so the blame for the faecal incontinence can be shifted from the child to faulty toiletting habits. The shame of the parents can also be alleviated by highlighting the biological reason for their child's problem. Effective treatment can only be achieved by education – fear or distaste of faeces often initiates the disastrous chain of events so difficult to reverse.

Relief of constipation Hospital admission is best sought so that the deconstipation exercise can be achieved, although the constipation clinic that Bennett (1988) has described has a high community involvement in the treatment. The contact between the practitioner and the patient must be maintained even during the hospital phase of the treatment. The deconstipation routine can be achieved by the use of phosphate enemas; micro-enemas; mineral oil or ducolax.

It is less important, however, to persevere with one of the above agents as long as the regime is successful. Once the bowel is clear (and this can be checked by comparing X-rays of 'before and after') the functioning of the bowel is maintained by tapering the medication over a few months and a toilet routine which allowes for twice daily sittings!

With this sort of approach it is useful to allow the patient some scope for decision making as this helps his self-esteem and increases the chances of compliance. Studies have shown (Levine and Bakow, 1976) that there are certain children who would be likely to have the least success in this type of therapy. If the client records the following in their history it is doubtful if the treatment will be successful:

A. Little stool retention at first.
B. Soiling at different times of the day.
C. Misbehaviour at school.
D. A blasé attitude about soiled underwear.

These children should be considered for early recall and referral to other specialists.

Habit training A second way of treating constipation-associated encopresis is to instigate a programme of habit training (Lowry, 1985). This involves the parents in much of the initial care. The bowel is cleared by the parents instilling a nightly enema. After this has been achieved the child should attempt to defeacate for 10 minutes after one or more meals. If the child fails at the end of the second day's attempts then an enema is again given, (eg, phosphate enemas).

This programme requires the parents to praise the child for successful bowel actions and accident free episodes while appearing fairly non-commital and calm about any incontinent episodes. The results achieved by such a programme are fairly impressive; over 50 per cent of the children become totally continent long-term with the number of incontinent episodes falling from 13.2 per week to 0.8 per week. Yet most encopretic children come from families where the stress level is extremely high and in such circumstances it may have been better to use a combination of recognised therapies such as structural family therapy and behaviour modification (Rydzinski and Kaplan, 1985).

By looking at the family as a cause of the child's disquiet and working on the areas of marital dispute and home-life disharmony that are causing the child's stress, great strides can be made in the treatment of this disturbing condition. Sharing the therapeutic tasks between husband and wife can often help to re-establish more balanced parental partnership towards the children. The couple together then can agree to be constant in their praise of the child when the desired behaviour is reached. This might be cold comfort to single parent families but it is often possible to involve other close friends of the family, or an older sibling might be prepared to help with the course of treatment.

Behaviour modification (Table 1) This can eliminate retentive encopresis very rapidly and has advantages over other methods of reducing the amount of parental involvement except for the integral praise for the desired behaviour. Despite the success of some of the

Treatments

References (continued)

Rydzinski, J.W. and Kaplans, L. (1985) A wolf in sheep's clothing? Simultaneous use of structural family therapy and behaviour modication in a case of encopresis and enuresis. *Human Sciences Press*, 71-81.

Schaefer, C.E. (1979) Childhood encopresis and enuresis: causes and theory. Van Nostrand Reinhold, New York.

Schmitt, B.D. (1984) Encopresis. *Primary Care*, **11**, 3, 497-511.

The Park Hospital for Children, Oxford (1986) Details of current therapy ideas and instructions to parents.

Wakefield, M.A. et al (1984) A treatment programme for faecal incontinence. *Developmental Medicine and Child Neurology*, **26**, 613-616.

Behaviour modification Three techniques can be used:

Gifts

The simplest of these is the giving of small gifts for unsoiled pants. This, however, has drawbacks in that it can encourage the child to become constipated to gain the desired gifts.

Overcorrection

This places a greater responsibility on the child, but still involves the giving of a gift. When the child soils he is required to wash out the soiled pants and 'practise' approaching the toilet from various directions and practise sitting on the toilet for a few seconds.

Negative reinforcement

By far the most successful technique experimentally, despite its apparent harshness:

1. After waking up, the child should sit on the toilet for 20 minutes or until a bowel action (whichever comes first).

2. Parental checks should be made every five minutes to ensure that the child remains on the toilet. The child is not allowed to do anything else on the toilet so he realises the purpose of the procedure. An effort can be made however to keep the child comfortably, for instance by supplying a stool on which to rest dangling feet. A bowel motion needs to be more, in bulk, than half a cup.

3. If no bowel action has occurred then the child has to stay on the toilet for 40 minutes after lunch or until a bowel action.

4. This procedure is then repeated following the evening meal for 90 minutes or until there is a bowel action. If the child has a bowel action, the daily pattern can be left for the rest of the day (Rolider van Houten, 1985).

Table 1. Behaviour modification.

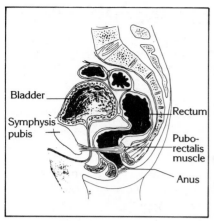

Figure 1. Position of bowel compared to other pelvic organs in the male.

Regime 1

Regime for the treatment of faecal incontinence –

Initial interview:
1st – Parents.
2nd – Parents and child.

Toileting regime:
Visits to the toilet after meals and before bed and improved diet.

Physiotherapy:
Abdominal massage.
Yoga exercises.
Hydrotherapy – helps the child to regain his or her confidence in public.
Play-therapy – useful when working with the under 5s.

Medication:
Success is regarded as:
  No soiling.
  Bowel actions.
  Regular.
  No laxatives.
  Maintained for 12 months.

Intimacy

Regime 2

Regime for management of retentive encopresis
1. Remove constipation by enemas, suppositories and laxatives.
2. Introduce a high-fibre diet.
3. Re-establish toileting regime.
4. Reduce anxiety and increase parental support for the child.

Regime for management of non-retentive encopresis
A. Encourage talk about the problem.
B. Restore confidence in the child.
C. Allow the child to decide when to go to the toilet.
D. Reward for staying clean.
  i Love and affection and extra time for games when in a non-soiled state works better than:
  ii Sweets and rewards.

(Schmitt, 1984)

---

above mentioned procedures, encopresis often requires a more detailed and integrated management philosophy so that the many strands of an individual's problem can be unravelled in a united professional way. An example of this unified approach has been developed by a team of doctors, social workers and physiotherapists from Aylesbury in Buckinghamshire (Wakefield, Woodbridge, Croke, Steward, 1984). Vital parts of this therapy are placed in the hands of the physiotherapists, teachers and play therapists to counteract the sort of natural peer revulsion and consequently damaged body-image of these encopretic children. An initial interview with the parents and child should be as informal as possible and although some practitioners like to see all the family together it may be an advantage to have the initial interview with the parents alone. It is often difficult to talk with a child present, and the value of a calm, reassuring first interview can be lost in the company of a distracting child. If the problem of the encopretic child is centred on a family-induced stress then this is often revealed at the first interview.

It is important to relieve as much anxiety as possible; diagrams (Figure 1) may help the child to understand the normal mechanisms of eliminating faeces. The child's often blasé attitude is explained as the most natural defence a child can employ given the seemingly unsolvable condition by which he is afflicted. An optimistic therapeutic climate must be maintained so that the most effective treatment can be pursued.

A toileting regime should be instigated with the help of the parents. A star chart helps to keep a track of the child's progress, but it is not considered important in its own right. Despite that, some children do become continent during this period. Physiotherapists can reteach defaecation techniques by allowing the child to rediscover the normal workings of his body. High fibre food is emphasised as being beneficial against the damaging effects of fast food (Regime 1).

The benefit of getting the child to be aware of his body is highlighted by the emphasis on massage, yoga and swimming. These previously forbidden activities (due to the fear of soiling in public) being now allowed, greatly assist the child in reducing anxiety while enhancing confidence and a state of wellbeing. Yoga exercises are designed to help muscle tone of the bowel (to prevent constipation) and to help the child relax. Each exercise sequence should be carried out daily at home (Park Hospital, 1986). The sequence should begin with a 'tummy rub' for five minutes.

This intimacy between child and parent often makes vast differences in the quality of their relationship and usually the stress that was a barrier to the improvement of the encopresis disappears. Several points need to be emphasised. First, teachers and other non-medical professionals may be ignorant about the reasons for faecal soiling. This may lead to situations where children are banned from school swimming lessons, even though no soiling has ever taken place in the pool and it may be just because the teacher in charge of the swimming lessons has been made aware of the child's condition. The therapist dealing with the case should endeavour to explain the condition to the relevant people. Much of this work could be undertaken by a nurse with access to the help of other professionals. However, encopresis is a multifaceted condition which needs the cooperation of a number of professional groups linked in a fairly formal way. Thankfully nearly all retentive encopresis disappears by the age of 16 years, while only one per cent of nonretentive encopresis has an organic background. This remaining 99 per cent also resolves itself by the age of adolescence.

The programme for retentive and nonretentive encopresis have been identified by Schmitt (1984) (Regime 2). As has been detailed above there are many therapeutic avenues open to the therapist to help solve encopresis. Pressure to create opportunities to extend help to these children and their families must be applied in areas without any facilities for the care of these children and their families.

Preventing Constipation and Faecal Incontinence in Children

Most children without physical and mental developmental difficulties will achieve continence of faeces by the age of four years. However, a few children do find it difficult, and most can be helpful at home. This handout will help you prevent your child having problems in achieving continence.

Babies

Babies are extremely sensitive to your reactions from a very early age, so it is a good idea not to show abhorrence towards a soiled nappy, however unpleasant it is to clean up.

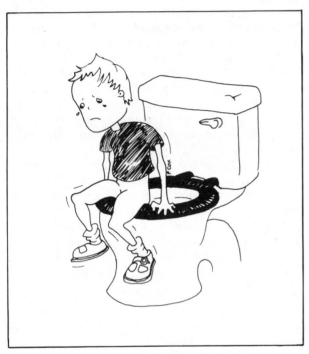

Children cannot produce much push if their feet are unsupported.

Words

The words you use to describe anything to do with faeces are also important. They should not carry any sort of negative implication. For example: 'Number two' is better than 'Poo', and 'Poo' is better than 'Dirty'.

Any family words for faeces are acceptable as long as they are not used in a negative sense for other things.

The potty

From about six months on (or when your child can sit up comfortably without help) it is useful to introduce the potty after feeding. This provides a comfortable seat to hold the child in the best position to catch the gut movement that happens after each meal. If your child learns to associate the potty with a pleasant, enjoyable time, it will be easier to achieve continence (musical potties that play a tune when used can help!)

One year old

After a year (seldom earlier) children may seem more conscious of their bowels, either by showing displeasure at a soiled nappy or by asking to sit on the potty. It is often worthwhile letting them go without nappies at certain times of the day (when convenient) with the potty near at hand, so they can practise skills of holding on.

Praise

Always make sure you praise your child when he or she is successful, but make sure you do not criticise any accidents.

Toilet

After potty training, the next stage is toilet training. It is a good idea to have an 'open door' toilet, so your child can see (and can therefore mimic) older children and adults using the toilet. A small toilet seat to fit over the bowl, and a stool to rest feet on will make the transition from potty to toilet much easier (though some children like the challenge of holding themselves on the toilet). Bottom wiping and hand washing can be taught at this stage.

Children who have become continent for some time can become incontinent again as a side effect of either stress and anxiety or constipation.

Stress

It is impossible to completely avoid stress and anxiety in childhood, but major episodes such as starting school, moving home or parental disharmony can result in loss of control. This is best prevented by preparing your child well in advance for any predictable changes in his or her life. Nothing can compensate for a warm, caring relationship with parents to minimise stress.

Constipation

This can usually be avoided by making sure your child eats plenty of fibre, drinks plenty of liquid and has time to defaecate without being rushed.

Faecal incontinence (encopresis) affects one or two children in every hundred, and can usually be completely resolved by the age of 16, but carries with it feelings of great revulsion. Careful handling while your child is developing continence can avoid problems later, as can efforts to avoid constipation.

If your child does have problems, your GP will be able to refer you to an expert in this condition. This might be another GP, a district nurse, health visitor, continence advisor or paediatrician. They will be able to set up a programme to help you and your child to solve the problem together.

Young schoolchildren given the use of a 'play hospital' and some education about hospitals and healthcare were found to be more knowledgeable and less fearful about the subjects.

Preparing children for hospital: a school-based intervention

Christine Eiser, BSc, PhD, *Research Fellow, Department of Psychology, University of Exeter*

Lesley Hanson, BA, RSCN, NVCert, *School Nursing Sister, Exeter Health Authority*

Hospital admission can be a frightening experience for children, particularly those who experience traumatic injury or sudden onset of chronic disease. To prepare them for the possibility of admission, it has been advocated that school-based education programmes be implemented (Elkins and Roberts, 1983; Peterson and Ridley-Johnson, 1983). This approach may also benefit children who are generally anxious about more routine visits to a doctor or dentist (Roberts et al, 1981).

One common approach to school-based intervention is the organised hospital tour. McGarvey (1983) reports that a programme for preschoolers, in which they were encouraged to "see, feel and experience" what happens in hospitals, was well received by children, teachers and parents. Three children who were subsequently hospitalised as emergency admissions were reported to adjust well.

An alternative technique involves setting up a 'play hospital' in school, and encouraging children to participate in both structured or free play situations (Brett, 1983). Elkins and Roberts (1984) set up a play hospital and used hospital volunteers dressed up as medical personnel to explain the equipment and procedures. The 25 children who took part in this activity subsequently reported fewer medical fears and were more knowledgeable about medical events than a control group of children.

Setting up a play hospital

This paper is concerned with our own experiences in setting up a play hospital in primary schools, and describing the children's responses. The purpose of the study was twofold: to increase children's hospital related knowledge, and reduce anxiety and fear. Since some of the children were quite young, we did not feel verbally based assessments, such as interviews or questionnaires, were appropriate as the main techniques for evaluation. Instead, we focused on qualitative changes in the nature of children's play. Groups of three children were videotaped playing with the equipment on two separate occasions, four weeks apart. During the intervening period, children were given the opportunity to handle and play with the equipment under the guidance of a school nurse and mother helpers. We hoped that, as a result of experience with the equipment and a range of educational activities, we would be able to identify changes in play, reflecting improved knowledge and attitudes towards hospitals and medical personnel.

Method

Subjects The children all attended a small first school (catering for five- to eight-year-olds) in a rural Devon town. There is little local industry, and unemployment is relatively high. The school, like most others in the district, caters for children predominantly from working and lower middle-class homes. None of the children suffered from any chronic condition, or had personal experience of hospital other than as an outpatient. Subjects were drawn from the reception class (five to 5½ years) and the third and fourth year (seven to eight years). They were collected from the classroom in groups of three (normally same-sex triads), selected by the teacher. Selection was random, rather than in terms of friendship patterns or ability levels. In all, 14 triads of five-year-olds and eight triads of eight-year-olds took part in the study.

Apparatus   A miniature hospital was set up in an empty classroom in the school. It was divided into four areas.

- The **reception** area consisted of a table and two chairs opposite each other. On the table was a telephone, notepad and pencil. There was also a display rack containing a selection of health education leaflets.
- The **hospital ward** consisted of two beds made with blankets, and a baby's cot, complete with doll. There was a food table on one of the beds, and a 'drip' hanging at the side. On a small table nearby were several pairs of rubber gloves, cotton facemasks and head covers (of the type used in surgery). On a series of open shelves was an array of medical equipment, including a stethoscope, syringe, tweezers, respiratory mask and nursing bowls.
- In the **X-ray** area was a hard table covered with a sheet. Above the table was a pretend light that could be swung through a semicircle, and two X-rays were hung on the wall.
- In the **surgery** areas, another hard table was covered by a sheet. There was also another green sheet on top, with a hole through which the 'surgery' could be performed. On nearby shelves were a number of surgical overalls, hats, masks, gloves and overshoes. In addition, there was a set of surgical equipment.

We also had a selection of dressing-up clothes: nursing uniforms of several grades (dark blue for sister, light blue for staff nurse, green for students); a doctor's white coat, and various 'patient' outfits – pyjamas, nighties and dressing-gowns.

Procedure

The 'hospital' was set up in a spare classroom. Children were brought into the hospital in groups of three, and invited to play with the equipment for 10 minutes. Over the following month, a number of activities were organised. The children were brought back to the hospital on several occasions, by the school nurse and mother helpers. On these occasions, some of the equipment was pointed out, and ward and surgical procedures explained. Other activities included a visit to the children's ward at the local hospital, and visits to the school from an ambulance and crew, health visitor and a guide dog and owner. Each class also undertook a health-related group project.

At the second filming, children were again brought to the 'hospital' in groups of three (as before) and told that this was their last opportunity to play with the equipment before it was moved to another school. Again, their play was videotaped during the 10-minute session.

Results

Area of activity   During the first play session, most groups of children focused all their activities on the ward area, with only two groups using the surgery and one using X-ray equipment. During the second session, all groups organised their play throughout all areas of the hospital. Games were more sequenced – patients were 'admitted' to the ward, and subsequently moved to X-ray and surgery, before being discharged.

Use of equipment   Children used a range of equipment at both sessions, although at first the stethoscope, syringe, bandages and masks were used considerably more than other pieces of equipment. During the second session, there was much greater use of all the equipment, with less emphasis on the stethoscope and syringe. There were also differences in how the children used the equipment. During the first session, play was often quite rough. Children were quite aggressive in the way they gave injections, for example. On the second occasion, all children were considerably more gentle, and apparently more aware of the impact of treatment on the patient. 'Patients' were therefore likely to be warned that an injection might hurt.

Acknowledgements
This work was funded by the Nuffield Foundation. We would like to thank Miss Joan Cudmore and the staff and children of Cowleymoor First School, Devon, and Philip Gurr for technical assistance. James Lang assisted with some of the children's interviews.

Does the play hospital work?

References

Azarnoff, P. (1982) Hospital tours for school children ended. *Pediatric Mental Health*, **1**, 2.

Brett, A. (1983) Preparing children for hospitalisation – a classroom teaching approach. *Journal of School Health*, **53**, 561-63.

Cradock, C., Cotler, S., Jason, L.A. (1978) Primary prevention: Immunisation of children for speech anxiety. *Cognitive Therapy and Research*, **2**, 389-396.

Elkins, R. and Roberts, M. (1983) Psychological preparation for pediatric hospitalisation. *Clinical Psychology Review*, **3**, 275-295.

Elkins, P. and Roberts, M. (1984) A preliminary evaluation of hospital preparation for nonpatient children: Primary prevention in a 'Let's pretend hospital'. *Children's Health Care*, **13**, 31-36.

Klingman, A., Melamed, B.G., Cuthbert, M.I., Hermecz, D.A. (1984) Effects of participant modelling on information acquisition and skill utilisation. *Journal of Consulting and Clinical Psychology*, **52**, 414-422.

McGarvey, M.E. (1983) Preschool hospital tours. *Children's Health Care*, **11**, 122-124.

Peterson, L. and Ridley-Johnson, R. (1980) Pediatric hospital response to survey a prehospital preparation for children. *Journal of Pediatric Psychology*, **5**, 1-7.

Peterson, L. and Ridley-Johnson, R. (1983) Prevention of disorders in children. In Walker, C.E. and Roberts, M.C. (Eds.) Handbook of Clinical Child Psychology. Wiley-Interscience, New York.

Roberts, M.C., Wurtele, S.K., Boone, R.R., Ginther, L.J., Elkins, P.D. (1981) Reduction of medical fears by use of modelling: A preventive application in a general population of children. *Journal of Pediatric Psychology*, **6**, 293-300.

Zastowny, T.R., Kirschenbaum, D.S., Meng, A.L. (1986) Coping skills training for children: Effects on distress before, during and after hospitalisation for surgery. *Health Psychology*, **5**, 231-247.

The handout overleaf can be photocopied for distribution to children being admitted to hospital.

'Healthcare staff' behaviour   There were substantial changes in the activities, particularly of nursing staff. During the first play session, nurses' activities involved care-taking, making beds, offering food and drink, or giving medicines. On the second, nurses spent a lot of time at the desk writing, or making phone calls. The role of the nurse seemed to have shifted from caretaker, to administrator!

Hospital atmosphere   On both occasions, children created an atmosphere of tension and emergency on the ward. Play invariably involved treating the very sick or dying, and speed and urgency characterised the interactions and conversations of staff.

Additional evaluations   All the children greatly enjoyed their time in the play hospital, and were keen to participate. Eleven children were interviewed in depth about their reactions to the project, and asked to describe what they had learned. All appeared to have benefitted substantially, both in terms of special information acquired, and in the development of non-fearful attitudes to hospital.

The ultimate justification for school-based preparation for hospitalisation may well be that children are less anxious and fearful about admission. There are, however, many practical difficulties involved in such an evaluation, particularly in that there may be a long interval between the intervention and admission, and that other mediating factors might then determine the child's behaviour. Such arguments have been put forward, and along with financial cuts, resulted in a reduction in these activities (Azarnoff, 1982). Certainly, the changes we identified were short-term, and we cannot speculate on the long-term value of our intervention.

Even within the short-term, however, we feel we can point to some increase in children's hospital-related knowledge. At the second session, children's play reflected greater awareness of a range of medical equipment, as well as knowledge of activities typical of admission, X-ray and surgery, and ward procedures.

There were also changes in hospital-related attitudes. The children seemed to have gained empathy with the patient's role; nurses were careful to warn patients of impending pain. In this respect, children seemed to have acquired very realistic appraisals of what happens in hospital. They were not only more aware of different equipment and techniques, but also aware of the potentially painful nature of medical treatment.

Perhaps more unfortunate was the change in children's perceptions of the nurse's role. During the first play session, 'nurses' cared for patients and tried to make them comfortable. On the second 'nurses' were preoccupied with administrative tasks, and had little, if any, time left for patient care. There also appeared to be greater awareness of a hierarchy among staff, with junior nurses being subordinate to more senior staff. To some extent, this kind of play may be closer to reality than that shown prior to the intervention, nevertheless, it seems somewhat regrettable.

Given the potential stress associated with hospitalisation (Peterson and Ridley-Johnson, 1980), it is important to develop a range of preparatory techniques for children. The school-based educational programme appears to have considerable merit, not least because it can be made available to all children before the need arises. It is not altogether clear at what level the programmes are successful; whether by increasing hospital related knowledge, reducing anxiety or helping the child develop skills to cope with hospital procedures. The success of the latter, described as 'stress-inoculation' procedures (Zastowny et al, 1986) in reducing stress in other situations (public-speaking [Cradock et al, 1978], and dental treatment [Klingman et al, 1984]), attests to the potential value of this approach in preparing children for hospitalisation.

At a practical level, the success of the play hospital is probably as dependent on the energy and enthusiasm of staff and children as on the particular contents. The overriding feeling of those who took part, however, both adults and children, was that the experience was worthwhile, and everyone learned a lot.

Going into Hospital

My name is ....

I am going to stay in .... **hospital**

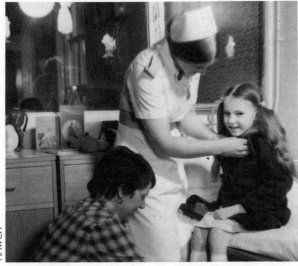

NAWCH

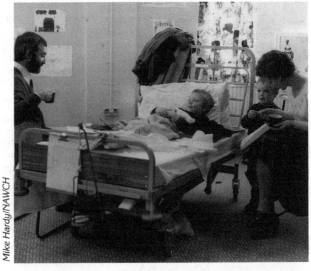

Mike Hardy/NAWCH

● When you go into hospital, there will be a lot of people there to look after you. Some of the nurses will stay awake all night, just in case you want them. The people who work in the hospital will make your food and give you everything you need, but your family and friends can visit you, and a grown-up can usually stay if you want them too.

● You will stay in a big room called a **ward,** which has big doors and windows, and there are always nurses there. The ward has lots of beds because there will be other children staying there as well as you. There will be a big bathroom with toilets nearby – a nurse will show you where it is.

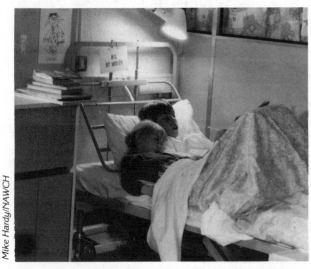

Mike Hardy/NAWCH

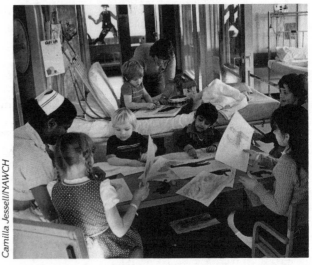

Camilla Jessell/NAWCH

● Your beds is on wheels, so you can be moved around on it. There are curtains that pull around, and a cupboard next to it. This cupboard is called a **locker,** and it is for you to keep your things in. You will also have a table, so you can eat or play while you are in bed.

● There is a playroom with a television and toys there for you to use.

Remember to bring your favourite toy, teddy bear or blanket with you when you come, so you don't miss it.

● Draw a picture of the ward with the beds, doors, windows, doctors, nurses, children and toys in it.

Practical aids and non-invasive therapy can help a family take the most significant step towards childhood continence by relieving anxiety

Bedwetting: The care of sufferers and families where there is nocturnal and diurnal enuresis

Arthur Turner, BA, RGN, DN, Cert
Community Liaison Officer, Newport, Gwent

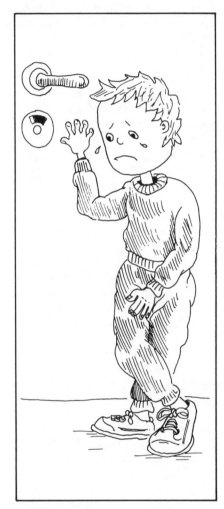

Bibliography
Parker, G. (1984) Incontinence services for the disabled child. *Health Visitor,* Article 1, **57,** 44-45. Article 2, **57,** 86-8.
Articles which highlight the need for expert domiciliary advice.
Nielsen, K.K. et al (1985) Value of cystourethroscopy in the assessment of children with recurrent urinary tract infections and/or enuresis. *Urology Research,* **13,** 137-9.
Research paper providing evidence of the lack of benefit from invasive investigation.
Family Services Unit, Discussion Paper (1982), Enuresis in School Children.
A booklet that carefully examines the despair and disruption enuresis can cause in socially impoverished families.

Controlling the urge to urinate can take many months for children to master and it seems quite reasonable for parents to tolerate accidents from their children right up to school age. Up to 15 per cent of children (Wille, 1986) who have delayed continence become continent spontaneously every year without any active treatment.

The absence of family anxiety is a sure way of bringing forward the time when the child is dry. However, many children and their parents begin to feel very anxious if the skill has not been mastered by the age of three, such is the apparent kudos of continent offspring. This stress can be increased by early school or younger children in the family who naturally increase the toil of washing and drying. Winter can seriously overburden even the most sophisticated washing and drying facilities and this may be the first reason for parents to seek help.

Diurnal enuresis is obviously far more difficult and embarrassing for the child than nocturnal enuresis; though between four and six years peer groups are not so cruel as they become later. There appears to be little treatment available before seven years, though a team of doctors from St James's University Hospital, Leeds, report some success using alarm procedures (Halliday, 1987).

There have been some promising results gained by the following non-invasive therapies:-

● Many children who wet themselves during the day appear to have functionally small bladders and a management programme that is designed to enlarge that functional size can be devised. Increasing the amount of drink the child has helps to increase the levels of urine produced and as long as this is accompanied by instructions to the child to resist the urge to urinate, initially for 10 seconds at the toilet edge and for increasing seconds daily, then this should have the effect of strengthening the resistance to the urge to urinate (Morgan, 1980).

  Similarly the child might be encouraged to go to the toilet every hour; a time interval that is lengthened by a quarter of an hour every week until the optimum is achieved.

● Hypnotherapy has recently been gaining favour amongst various professional groups dealing with children. Medically qualified hypnotherapists can give an expert service as young children are particularly susceptible to this deep relaxation. A tape of instructions can be played as the young child first falls asleep. This may not be immediately effective but often the fact that a solution is being sought can go some way to relieving parental anxiety. It is often said that the anxious parents require treatment first!

Children and their families often need practical support and this can take the form of offering mattress covers or making the parents aware of what type of help is available (Children's Society, 1986).

It is of some concern that children as young as four are subject to drug therapy which is of limited use but has potentially fatal side effects.

Imipramine syrup has been cited as the most common fatal overdose in the under five age group, often through siblings drinking the bedwetter's medicine. Viloxazine seems to work as effectively as Imipramine but with fewer side-effects (Attenburrow, Stanley and Holland, 1984). An anti-diuretic agent such as Desmospressin (DDAVP) taken as a snuff, while not being recommended as a first choice treatment, has some value as a safe drug with rapid effect, particularly for 'one-off' situations (Wille, 1986).

Treatment options

References

Attenburrow, A.A., Stanley, T.V. and Holland, R.P.C. (1984) Nocturnal enuresis; a study. *The Practitioner*, **228**, 99.

Azrin, N.H., Sneed, T.J. and Foxx, R.M. (1974) *Behaviour, Research and Therapy*, **12**, 147-56.

Blumenthal, I. Nocturnal Enuresis (Bedwetting); A Guide for Parents. Eastwood and Son Limited, London.

Bugge-Nielsen, J., Norgaard, J.P. and Djurhuus, J.C. (1985) *Urology*, **XXVL**. 316-9.

Halliday, S. (1987) Successful management of daytime enuresis using alarm procedures: a random controlled trial. *Archives of Disease in Childhood*, **62**, 132-7.

Maizels, M. and Firlit, C.F. (1986) Guide to the history of enuretic children. *American Family Physician*, **33**, 4, 205-9.

Maizels, M. and Rossenbaum, D. (1985) Successful treatment of nocturnal enuresis: a practical approach. *Primary Care*, **12**, 4, 621-35.

Morgan, R. (1980) Childhood Incontinence. Disabled Living Foundation; Heinemann Medical Books Limited, London.

Norton, C. (1986) 'Incontinence in Childhood'. Nursing for Continence. Beaconsfield Publishers Limited, Buckinghamshire.

Norgaard, J.P., Pedersen, E.B. and Djurhuus, J.C. (1985) Diurnal anti-diuretic hormone levels in enuretics. *The Journal of Urology*, **134**, 1029-31.

O'Regan, S. and Yazbeck, S. (1985) Constipation: A cause of enuresis, urinary tract infection and vesico-urethral reflux in children. *Medical Hypothesis* **17**, 409-13.

Taylor, P.D. and Turner, R.K. (1975) A clinical trial of continuous, intermittent and overlearning bell and pad techniques for nocturnal enuresis. *Developmental, Medical and Child Neurology*, **13**, 281-93.

The Children's Society (1986) Submission to the Social Work Committee.

Wells, S.A. (1984) Project for ENB Course 978.

Wille, S. (1986) Comparison of desmopression and enuresis alarm for nocturnal enuresis. *Archives of Disease in Childhood*, **61**, 30-3.

(Attenburrow, Stanley and Holland, 1984). Secondly, some general practitioners are still advising that children should be deprived of fluids for up to four hours before they go to bed despite the clear evidence that this antagonises the situation (Wells, 1984).

Various suggestions have been made as to why enuresis should be such a common problem. Many medical experts have cited a small bladder capacity as being primarily responsible for bedwetting (Norgaard, Pedersen and Djurhuus, 1985) in that this small functional capacity is overwhelmed at night by a lack of diurnal rhythms in anti-diuretic hormones. Norgaard had also suggested that enuresis might act as a safety valve against the possibility of reflux nephropathy (Bugge-Nielsen, Norgaard and Djurhuus, 1985). Constipation has been implicated by O'Regan (O'Regan et al, 1985) and it seems logically linked to other theories, as a faecal mass will reduce functional bladder capacity. Another popular assertion is that a child wets him/herself during deep sleep, this has, however been largely disproved by the work of Norgaard, though many parents say their children are unrousable (Norgaard, Pederson and Djurhuus, 1985). Medical tests such as Urodynamics and Cysto-urethroscopy does not appear to have any tangible benefits as the results do not have any effect on the choice of treatment.

Many parents restrict the child's drinks hours before bed but this, as previously indicated is counterproductive. 'Lifting' the child may well be convenient for the parents and can prevent the daily chore of wet beds. This is a good method of early control as long as it is tailed off before the child becomes used to the nightly intervention. As the child becomes more aware, it would be better to vary the time of 'lifting' and to provide a potty near the bed, plus a night light so that the child is confident about getting up in the night.

However, the mainstay of all treatment remains the buzzer/alarm. This has a very good response rate but if the management of the therapy is poor and haphazard then the relapse rate can be as high as 40 per cent (Wille, 1986). As there is a natural rate of continence acquisition then it is a good idea to spend the first treatment meetings undertaking a complete assessment (Maizel and Firlitt, 1986). The general practitioner should have regard to urinary infections and constipation, while the practitioner caring for the enuretic child should take into account the wider social implications (See Table 1).

The two mat buzzer with a durable box remains the first choice, though the single mat version appears to have the considerable advantage of being easy to use it is also more flimsy (Eastleigh Model SM1 — 1986). Practical experience indicates that the small body-worn type of buzzer is too insubstantial for general use. However, it is essential that the therapist shows the family how to use whichever type of buzzer is available, if necessary in the home situation. Advice such as avoiding nylon sheets, not restricting fluids unduly and maintaining a calm and encouraging attitude needs constant re-emphasising (Norton, 1986).

Once dryness has been achieved it may well be very useful to try a technique called 'overlearning'. This merely asks for the child to drink extra fluids before bed. Usually this precipitates more wetting at night but eventually the dry period returns and the relapse rate is considerably reduced (Blumenthal, 1983). Intermittent reinforcement using the buzzer at intervals *after* the dry period of 14 nights has been achieved, seems to protect the child against relapse while use of the buzzer, as soon as the relapse occurs, also quickly returns the dry pattern (Taylor and Turner, 1975).

A technique called 'dry-bed training' described by Azrin, Sneed and Foxx 1974, (See Table 2 page 49), should be reserved for very highly motivated children and their families. It is a strenuous form of therapy which requires at least one all-night session of training. Its attractions are that it has the lowest of all relapse rates, yet I feel it is too daunting for most families (The Children's Society, 1986).

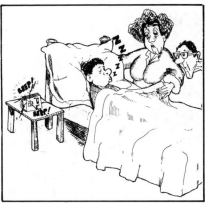

The buzzer/alarm is the mainstay of all treatment.

Health Authorities need to ensure that services for the incontinent child and his/her family are well integrated, well organised, open to all sufferers and monitored by staff who have been well trained in alternative therapies and who show a compassionate attitude to therapy.

Table 1. Examples of the type of questions needed to be answered in the assessment of the enuretic child (Maizels and Rosenbaum, 1985).

(1) Were there any pre-birth problems and was the birth itself long and traumatic?

(2) Have there been any significant childhood problems? The period between 3-4 years old is a very sensitive one and secondary bedwetting (primary being enuresis that has never resolved) can occur in previously continent children in response to a traumatic event.

(3) Which type of toilet training was used?
Strict toilet training can have marked effects as the children develop.

(4) What is their pattern of micturition?
It is very important to gain a detailed history.

(5) What is their pattern of voiding?
It is equally important to gain a concise pattern.

(6) Does the child have a urinary infection?
This can often make the enuresis worse or be a sign, especially in repeated chronic urinary infections, of a more serious problem in the urinary system.

(7) What is the child's bowel pattern?
Constipation can exacerbate urinary incontinence.

(8) Are there other external problems around the perineum?
Congenital abnormalities can sometimes be missed.

(9) Do they suffer from food allergies and sensitivities?
Caffeine (also in 'Pepsi'), milk and tartrazine have been implicated in the causation of nocturnal enuresis and diurnal frequency.

(A) Intensive training — one night

One hour before bed time
(1) Child informed of training procedure in detail.
(2) Buzzer is placed on the bed.
(3) Positive toiletting practice (20 trials).
- Child lies on bed.
- Child counts to 50.
- Child arises and attempts to urinate in the toilet.
- Child goes back to bed.
- Repeat all steps 20 times.

At bed time
- Child has a drink.
- Child repeats instructions to the trainer.
- Child goes to bed.

Hourly awakenings
- Slight prompt to awaken child.
- Child walks to bathroom.
- At bathroom door and before urination child is asked to inhibit urination for one hour. (for children over 6 years). If child unable to inhibit urination:
  (a) Child urinates in the toilet.
  (b) Receives praise from teacher.
  (c) Child returns to bed.
- At bedside *child* feels the bed sheets and comments on their dryness.
- Child receives praise for dry bed.
- Child is given a drink.
- Child goes back to sleep.

Procedure when an accident occurs
- Trainer disconnects the buzzer.
- Trainer awakens the child and tells him off for wetting the bed.
- Trainer directs child to toilet to finish off urination.
- Child is given cleanliness training.
  (a) Child is required to change night clothes.
  (b) Then the child removes the wet sheet and places it with dirty laundry.
  (c) Trainer re-engages the buzzer.
  (d) Child gets clean sheets and remakes the bed.
- The child has to practise the positive toiletting a further 20 minutes and before going to bed the next evening.

(B) Post-training supervision (the following night after training begins)

Before bedtime
- Buzzer placed on the bed.
- Positive toiletting practice (only if accident occurred the previous night).
- Child is reminded of the need to keep dry (and to undertake the cleanliness training and positive toiletting if wet the previous evening).
- The child repeats the parent's instructions.

Night time toiletting
- At the parent's bedtime awake the child and send him to the toilet.
- After each dry night the child should be awakened 30 minutes earlier.
- Awakening should be discontinued when the awakening is within one hour of the child's bedtime.
- When accidents occur the child receives cleanliness training and positive toiletting practice immediately following wetting and at bedtime the next day.

After a dry night
- Both parents praise the child for not wetting the bed.
- Parents praise the child at least five times during the day.
- Child's favourite adults are encouraged to praise him.

(C) Normal routine (after seven consecutive dry nights)
- Buzzer no longer placed on the bed.
- Parents inspect the bed each morning.
  (a) If wet the child receives cleanliness training *immediately* and positive toiletting the following evening.
  (b) The child is praised for a dry bed.
- If two accidents occur within one week then post training supervision begins again.

Bedwetting (Nocturnal enuresis)

Bedwetting occurs in all babies until about eighteen months of age. There is simply not enough maturity in the nerves and the brain for the desire to urinate to be stopped until a suitable receptacle can be found.

Many parents use a potty in order to mimic continence in the early months and there seems little wrong with this approach so long as there is no stress involved with the process. Sitting on a potty may be a peaceful time of the day enabling the parents to read and play with the child. Praise for the desired result, (ie urine in the potty) will effectively begin to shape the child's behaviour. As the child matures he/she will gradually learn to hold onto urine until voiding is permitted in the socially acceptable place, (ie potty/toilet).

However, it is quite normal for children of three-and-a-half to still be wetting the bed (25 per cent at least) and accidents can continue to occur for a number more years. Anxieties in the child's life (such as a new baby/death of a relative) can return the bedwetting to previously continent children.

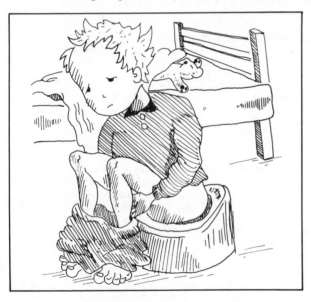

Normally, children will begin to have dry nappies in the morning indicating that the bladder capacity is increasing. The child may wake up in order to urinate (albeit sometimes too late) and at this stage it is often worth leaving a potty in the bedroom with a small light nearby. This can encourage the child to be independent.

'Lifting' the child when the parents go to bed does seem to work but it is as well to do so at varying times in the late evening rather than at the same time each night so the child does not rely on this lifting. Encourage the child to drink a reasonable amount of fluids *during the whole day*. Excessive drinks will lead to incontinence at night but *heavily restricting fluids does not* help at all, indeed usually makes the problem worse. This is because restricted fluid intake creates a small bladder and therefore one that cannot hold sufficient urine until morning.

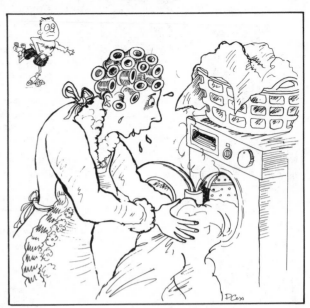

Only limited treatment can be given to children before the age of seven years (eight years in boys) as a younger child is considered unlikely to be able to give sufficient cooperation in following the necessary instructions.

Holding practice can help to enable the child's bladder to hold more urine. This involves the child counting to ten at the edge of the toilet before passing urine. It can also involve *gradually* lengthening the time between visits to the toilet.

Additives in the diet have often been implicated in bedwetting especially those in orange squash and cola drinks. It is a good idea to encourage the child to drink diluted pure fruit juice instead. Treatment options include:

Support for the family
Usually from the health visitor, as between the ages of three and seven spontaneous improvement often occurs without any therapy.

Advisors to help
Professionals likely to be involved:

General Practitioner.
Specialist Health Visitor.
Health Visitor.
School Nurse.
District Continence Advisor.
Social Worker.
Community Medical Officer.
Medical Consultant in Child Health.
Clinical Psychologist.
Family Counselling.
Medical Hypnotherapist.

It is usual for just one of the above agencies to maintain contact with the child and family while using the other experts as referral points. Too many people can lead to confusion and anxiety.

A star chart

Although not a therapy in itself it does help many younger children who benefit from 'winning' gold stars for a sequence of dry nights.

A dot-to-dot plus grab-bag

This technique involves drawing a large dot-to-dot of the child's favourite toy which can be bought at the completion of the dots. For each dry night the child completes a dot. Every fifth dot is larger and rewarded by a 'grab-bag' in which a number of smaller treats are attainable.

Treatment for a urine infection

Urine infection can make the bedwetting much worse and needs to be treated. This treatment is prescribed by a doctor following a simple test.

Treatment for constipation

Constipation can make bedwetting a lot worse and the treatment will include a change of diet to one that contains a lot of roughage/fibre.

Buzzer

The buzzer is usually central to most treatments. It is often available from the Health Authorities but can be loaned from the manufacturers (N.H. Eastwood & Son Limited, 70 Nursery Road, London, N14 5QH). To ensure that the treatment is successful and permanent three techniques have been developed to be used with the buzzer:-

1. Overlearning

Where after 14 dry nights extra fluid is drunk last thing at night to ensure the increased capacity of the bladder.

2. Intermittent reinforcement

After 14 dry nights any lapse is treated with the buzzer for a further week.

3. Dry bed training

This is a highly intensive treatment which needs great motivation but has very good and often permanent results.

Hypnotherapy

This is the teaching of deep relaxation which can eliminate the stress that perpetuates the bedwetting.

Drug therapy

This has to be prescribed by a doctor and there are a number of different drugs which can be used.

Treatments may well be offered in a different sequence depending on the individual problems the child presents with and the personal preference of the person organising the treatment.

If a buzzer is used it will be fully explained by the clinic specialist and she should show how to place the buzzer in the bed in which it is to be used. Simple advice will be given to improve the chances

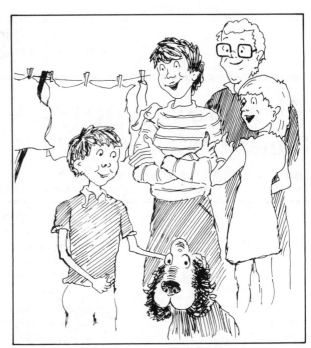

of treatment success; for example cotton sheets are better than nylon. In some Health Authorities a laundry service might be available and a DHSS grant might be given towards the purchase of extra linen.

While it is not usual to supply mattress covers the Health Authority can do so in cases of hardship and the Department of Health and Social Security are able to give awards in particular cases towards the purchase of new mattresses; especially those families on Supplementary Benefit.

Above all it is important for both the families and children suffering from bedwetting to be aware that it is quite normal. One in 14 at the age of 11 is still wet at night and therefore within an average class there are probably two or three bedwetters. Second, a fifth of these children become dry spontaneously every year so there is a good chance that your child will do so whatever treatments are tried.

Smaller devices are now used, with success, that attach to the child's pyjamas whilst some urine sensitive receptors are placed in a small pad worn between the legs. Although it may seem that the buzzer will not be successful where children share a bedroom or there are other practical problems, it is often the case that there is a solution. Ask your clinic specialist for advice on how to overcome these difficulties.

Remember

1. The child is not bedwetting deliberately.
2. Two or three children in each lower secondary school class are likely to be bedwetters.
3. One in five children will become dry without any treatment.
4. The child needs loving support and encouragement, not punishment.
5. Punishment will only make the problem worse.

Temper tantrums, learning difficulties, anxiety, aggression
. . . all are clinical features of childhood hyperactivity. But can
they be alleviated by altering the diet in some way?

The hyperactive child:
Dietary management?

John W.T. Dickerson, PhD, FIBiol, FIFST, FRSH
Formerly Professor of Human Nutrition, Department of Biochemistry, University of Surrey, Guildford

The idea that behaviour disorders might be caused by food is not new. As long ago as 1945, Schneider suggested that 'allergy' played an important role in causing childhood hyperkinesis. Current interest in the possible role of diet in the aetiology of behavioural disorders stems largely from the suggestion by the late Dr B.F. Feingold that approximately 30 to 50 per cent of hyperactive children show a significant improvement in behaviour when placed on a special elimination programme (see Feingold, 1975). Feingold's work suggested that naturally occurring salicylates and artificial food additives may cause hyperkinesis in children with a genetically determined predisposition. Feingold's observations were extended to children with disruptive behaviour associated with learning disability, epilepsy and mental handicap. It is not surprising that these observations have caused concern to food manufacturers and particularly parents of such children, who began to see in this industry and the complexity of food the cause of their children's problems.

What is hyperkinesis?

The terms hyperactivity, hyperkinesis and hyperkinetic syndrome are used loosely in both medical and lay literature. Clinical features include overactivity, inattentiveness, distractibility, poor tolerance of frustration, temper tantrums, impulsive behaviour, resistance to discipline, anxiety, aggression, cognitive dysfunction and learning problems. In some children the disorder is associated with epilepsy or some other neurological disorder and in America in particular children are often described as having 'minimal brain dysfunction'.

In the UK, the 'hyperkinetic syndrome' has been reported to occur in 0.1 per cent of children (Rutter et al, 1970), whereas in the US it is said to be present in four to 10 per cent of all school-age children. This difference is probably due to the criteria of diagnosis. From its very nature it is clear that psychosocial factors may be responsible for the condition. It is all too easy for parents and teachers to ignore this possibility and look for dietary or other factors to account for a child's unruly behaviour. Some of these children may be very intelligent and are simply frustrated.

Aetiology

Many factors have been suspected or presumed to play a role in the aetiology of hyperkinesis. Complications during pregnancy, smoking during pregnancy, genetic factors, environmental pollutants (particularly lead from car exhaust fumes), adverse reactions to foods, disturbances in the metabolism of the cerebral neurotransmitters dopamine and noradrenalin, as well as disturbances in parental-child interrelationships, have all been implicated. It is unfortunate, but not altogether unreasonable, that doctors faced with a child with this sort of problem may all too readily prescribe drugs, particularly amphetamine, methyl phenidate (Ritalin) and tricyclic antidepressants, with or without behaviour modifications, in attempting to treat the disorders. These treatments, particularly by the drugs, while ameliorating symptoms, do nothing to remove the cause of the hyperactivity. The possibility of undesirable side-effects cannot be ruled out.

Diagnosis

If a child is obviously hyperactive, attempting to identify the factors responsible may seem a forbidding, time-consuming task to which busy doctors feel unable to devote sufficient time. A nurse working in the community can make a substantial contribution in obtaining the necessary information for an accurate diagnosis. By visiting parents in their homes, and where appropriate, talking to teachers at school, she can help to obtain the necessary comprehensive appraisal of medical, social, educational and psychological factors (Varga, 1979). Typically, the child will have a history of abnormalities in the key temperamental traits mentioned above. It is important to determine how long the child has had symptoms. It has been suggested (Rutter et al, 1970) that 'hyperkinetic syndrome' be used only for children whose symptoms arise before the age of five years.

As infants (Weiss and Hechtman, 1979), hyperactive children may have been poor and irregular sleepers, and have had colic and feeding problems. Sometimes infants that develop hyperactivity have not enjoyed being held for more than a few minutes. Hyperactive toddlers are described as children who never walk but run, do not play with one object for more than a few seconds and who combine an impulsive behaviour with a lack of fear. When the child reaches three to four years parents complain that he is very demanding, does not listen and finds it difficult to play with other children. Parents despair that neither praise nor punishment is effective, that 'nothing works'. Not infrequently, parents will disagree as to what methods are most helpful.

It is not surprising that hyperactive children present considerable problems to teachers. Their behaviour will not only have a marked disruptive effect on class discipline but also lead to the underachieving of intellectual potential. If the child is naturally intellectually very 'bright', problems at school, as in the home, may be due largely to frustration.

It is only after all this information has been properly assessed attempts can be made to diagnose the cause of the child's behaviour problems.

Food and hyperactivity

The idea that food may be the cause of a child's difficult behaviour is attractive. It is something tangible that parents can understand and, theoretically, if the foods can be found and eliminated from the diet, the child should be better. The satisfactory testing of Feingold's hypothesis that a considerable amount of hyperactivity in children is caused by foods containing salicylates and additives, particularly colours, has proved difficult; reported studies are open to severe criticism with reference to the diagnosis and description of the children's condition, placebo control and dosage of additives (Rippere, 1983). It is difficult to accept that they provide a satisfactory basis for the confident statement by the US Nutrition Foundation that they ''provide sufficient evidence to refute the claim that artificial flavourings and natural salicylates produce hyperactivity''. There may be a real 'danger' inherent in the Feingold approach (Rippere, 1983) in that if omission of all food additives and salicylates is found not to result in improved behaviour it may be concluded that food is not the cause of the condition. The possibility must always be considered that any food may cause hyperactivity in a susceptible child.

There is a widespread belief that sugar (sucrose) causes behaviour and learning problems in children. These have been attributed to reactive hypoglycaemia or 'allergic' reaction. However, both these hypotheses remain at present untested and unproven (Ferguson et al, 1986). However, in relation to individual children, it may be prudent to retain an open mind on this matter because some children do like large amounts of sugar, which may be associated with hyperactive and aggressive behaviour in some.

Hyperactive Children's Support Group

The Hyperactive Children's Support Group (HACSG) has done much in the UK to help families with hyperactive children. It provides a list of foods suitable for hyperactive children which are salicylate- and additive-free (page 96). They also provide ideas for nutritious meals. A survey by questionnaire (Higgs, Colquhoun and Dickerson, unpublished) of 117 hyperactive children who had adopted the HACSG dietary programme showed that parents of over 90 per cent of the children claimed improvements in coordination, concentration, fits or tantrums and aggressiveness; over 50 per cent for crying or screaming; 82 per cent in speech; 73 per cent in disruptive behaviour; and 71 per cent in self-abuse. These results confirmed those of a previous study which had involved over 100 other children (Pepler, Colquhoun and Dickerson, unpublished). Taken together, these studies appear to offer support for the Feingold hypothesis. However, considerable caution is needed in their interpretation. First, they were obtained by questionnaire and it is very difficult to construct an unbiased questionnaire, particularly when parents are reporting on their children. Furthermore, the sample of parents who completed the questionnaire may well have been self-selected with mainly those parents who thought their children had benefited from the diet being willing to complete it. The new diet could have been a considerable nutritional improvement on the child's normal diet and the changes therefore have been due to improvements in general nutrition.

Furthermore, the possibility must be considered that putting the children on the diet resulted in an improvement in parent-child relationships, with the parents taking rather more interest in their children. However, bearing all these difficulties in interpretation in mind, it can be recommended with some confidence that parents of hyperactive children try the diet. It is nutritious, harmless, a good diet for all the family and might help to cure hyperactivity even though the precise reason for the improvement cannot be defined.

A more recent study (Egger et al, 1985) has confirmed that foods other than those suggested by Feingold can cause hyperactivity. In this study, 76 selected overactive children were treated with an oligoantigenic diet consisting of two meats (eg, lamb and chicken), two carbohydrate sources (eg, potatoes and rice), two fruits (eg, banana and apple), vegetable (eg, any brassica), water, calcium (calcium gluconate 3g/day) and vitamins (Abidec 0.6ml/day). The diet was adjusted to suit the taste and habits of the family, and to avoid any foods suspected of causing symptoms and those for which the child had a particular like or craving. A total of 42 children improved; of these, 21 recovered completely and achieved a normal range of behaviour. The results were confirmed in 28 other children by a double-blind, crossover, placebo-controlled trial in which foods thought to provoke symptoms were reintroduced. A total of 48 foods were incriminated. While artificial food colours and preservatives were the commonest provoking substances, no child was sensitive to these alone. The sensitivity of children to very specific foods is illustrated by the finding that sugar provoked a change in behaviour in nine of 55 children tested.

The nurse's role

Parents of hyperactive children need help, understanding and reassurance. A trusted community nurse or health visitor may be the best person to provide this, but she will work as part of a team. The extent of her role will depend on the child's doctor, the availability of dietetic advice and, of course, her own knowledge and interest. Doctors are not always sympathetic to parents who consult them about overactive children. In such cases it may be that a health visitor can pursue the matter herself by collecting the information on which a diagnosis can be based. In addition to their behaviour, information should be obtained about the child's usual diet and in particular any likes or cravings for specific foods.

All community nurses and health visitors should have sufficient knowledge to detect nutritional inadequacy in a child's diet, but if possible the matter should be discussed with a dietitian. If it is decided to proceed with an investigation of the child for reactions to specific foods, again this is best done with the help of a dietitian, with the nurse having an intermediary caring and supporting role. It is essential that testing is done as objectively as possible; a nurse in touch with the family in the home can be a great help in this. False positive reactions are often recorded. Careful testing can seem tedious but is essential if anxious parents are to be prevented from putting a child on an unnecessarily restricted diet in the hope of a 'cure'. It should not be forgotten that sometimes the cause of the problem is the parents' own behaviour towards the child.

References

Egger, J., Carter, C.M., Graham, P.J. et al (1985) Controlled trial of oligoantigenic treatment in the hyperkinetic syndrome. *Lancet*, **1**, 540-5.

Feingold, B.F. (1975) Hyperkinesis and learning disabilities linked to artificial food flavours and colours. *American Journal of Nutrition*, **75**, 797-803.

Ferguson, H.B., Stoddart, C. and Simen, J.G. (1986) Double blind challenge studies of behavioural and cognitive effects of sucrose-aspartame ingestion in normal children. *Nutritional Reviews*, **44**, 144-58.

Rippere, V. (1983) Food additives and hyperactive children. A critique of Conners. *British Journal of Clinical Psychology*, **22**, 19-32.

Rutter, M., Tizard, J. and Whitmore, K. (1970) Education, Health and Behaviour. Longman, London.

Schneider, W.F. (1945) Psychiatric evaluation of the hyperkinetic child. *Journal of Pediatrics*, **26**, 559-70.

Varga, J. (1979) The hyperactive child. *American Journal of Diseases of Childhood*, **133**, 413-8.

Weiss, G. and Hechtman, L. (1979) The hyperactive child syndrome. *Science*, **205**, 1348-53.

Diet and Hyperactive Children
Foods suitable for hyperactive children

Any cereals without artificial colouring and flavouring

All homemade bakery goods and sweets

Bakery goods preferably made with 81-100% stoneground flours – plain or self-raising

Shop-bought brown bread made from 81-100% stoneground flour

All fresh meats, offal, poultry, and white fish

Homemade ice cream, sweets, lollies, jellies made with permitted fruit juices

Plain gelatin for jellies

Bananas

Lemons

Grapefruit

Pears   } Permitted as fruits and juices

Pineapple

Melon

Avocado pears

Homemade lemonade

Homemade or shop jam with permitted fruits but without artificial colouring and flavouring

Pure honey

Homemade puddings

Plain yoghurt

'7 up' drink

Milk, eggs, white cheeses and unsalted butter

Pure cooking oils and fats

White vinegar

All fresh vegetables

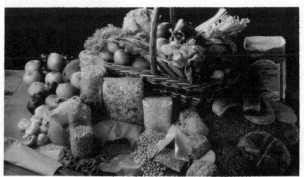

Photo courtesy of BDA.

Points to remember if your child if hyperactive

1. Overactivity is a complex condition. It can be caused by a number of factors, including environmental pollutants such as lead, and foods.

2. It is worth trying to identify the cause of your child's behaviour problem because if this is avoided your child could be much better.

3. You will need help if you are trying to investigate the problem. You should discuss the matters with your doctor and ask if it is possible to see a health visitor or dietitian.

4. In order to help your doctor, keep a record of your child's behaviour and of his diet for three weeks.
   Especially note those things that are eaten frequently and those consumed between meals, such as ice lollies and coloured drinks.

5. Discuss the record with your doctor and/or health visitor.

6. You may be advised to submit your child to tests. The only tests that are worth considering are those that involve the elimination of certain foods from the diet. Other tests, such as skin tests or blood tests are unreliable.

7. Try to change to a diet based on wholefoods. The one suggested by the Hyperactive Children's Support Group is worth trying.

8. Keep in touch with your health visitor.

Useful address: Hyperactive Children, 150 Donvant Road, Killay, Swansea. Telephone: 0792 201749. Offers information and advice.

Many nurses come into contact with families suffering from sleep disruption caused by babies and young children. Here, the identification and prevention of some common sleep problems are looked at.

Silent Nights

Marjorie Keys, RGN, HVCert, DipHV
Health Visitor, Cupar, Fife

The idea of 'good sleeping patterns' is obviously subjective – what one parent considers to be a good pattern may be unacceptable to another. Similarly, the term 'sleeping problem' is difficult to define, as it depends entirely on the parents' perception of the situation – they must decide for themselves if a problem exists for them. Perhaps a good sleeping pattern is best described as one which fits in with the customs and needs of the rest of the family and avoids disruption of the parents' sleep during the night.

Studies have shown that sleeping difficulties are one of the commonest problems experienced by parents of young children. John and Elizabeth Newson (1965) found, in a study of 700 one-year-olds in Nottingham, that 35 per cent of mothers had been woken by their babies on the night before the interview. Interviewing mothers of four-year-old children, they found that 20 per cent still woke at night, some only once or twice a week, but some much more frequently (Newson and Newson, 1970). In 1968, Seiler, a Scottish GP set out to examine the prevalence of sleep problems in children aged between six months and five years. He found that in his survey of 234 children, 40 per cent had been a sleep problem at some time.

In my own health visiting practice, a close examination of visits during a recent typical four-week period, shows that sleeping disturbances are a frequently mentioned problem. During this period, sleeping difficulties were expressed at over one third of my visits (see Table 1).

| | Age | | |
	0 – 1	1 – 5	Total
Total child/visits	38	35	73
Problem*:-			
Sleeping*	16	11	27
Feeding*	11	4	15
General Health*	9	5	14
Behaviour	0	6	6

*Problem indicates difficulty expressed, however slight. Parents were asked specifically about each of these topics. Two children in a household counted as two visits. Where more than one problem mentioned, recorded in all relevant columns.

Table 1. Visits to families with children under five years in a four week period.

Sleep cycles and their relevance

Since research into sleep first started in 1952, a standard language for describing different levels of sleep has evolved, and sleep is said to have two forms – orthodox and rapid eye movement (REM) 'dreaming' sleep. Orthodox sleep has four stages, from light sleep which is easily roused to almost total oblivion. Adults spend about 80 per cent of their time in deep sleep but babies less, and we all go through the four stages of sleep several times each night. One full sleep cycle, known as the ultradian rhythm, takes about 100 minutes in adults, but only about 50 minutes in infants (Haslam, 1984).

Babies, like the rest of us, are most prone to wakening during stage 1 sleep. If a baby then requires the help of a parent to get back to sleep, parents may be disturbed several times a night and are likely to be often woken from deep sleep.

Effects on the parent

The effects on the rest of the family can be insidious and near-catastrophic. A baby or child with a 'sleeping problem' will almost always catch up on the required sleep the next day, but for many parents this is impossible. Although studies may show that adults can survive on remarkably little sleep (Horne, 1981), an exhausted mother who has no expectation of ever getting enough sleep can find life unbearable. She becomes short-tempered with the whole family, has no energy for anything but the most basic tasks, loses interest in her marriage and in outside activities and often loses self-esteem, particularly if she feels the sleeping problem is her fault. Worst of all, the resentment felt towards her baby in the middle of the night can spill over into the daytime hours, and she may indeed begin to hate her child more than she loves him.

Parents in this situation often resort to giving the wakeful child literally anything he demands in the middle of the night, so that they can all get some sleep. Babies may be given several bottles of milk a night; toddlers brought downstairs to play in the early hours of the morning; children allowed to force parents out of their own bed. Often, parents are unaware that other families are suffering a similar fate and feel ashamed of their inability to cope. Surprisingly often they do not ask for help and during my own visits I have found there is sometimes no disclosure of sleeping problems until the parents are specifically asked how their child sleeps at night. They may then describe the most appalling difficulties which have hitherto gone unmentioned.

A problem solved?

Helping parents who are suffering from disturbed sleep can be a great challenge. Some are so desperate they will agree to try almost anything, while others may be afraid of making a bad situation even worse. Sometimes there seems no reason for the wakefulness, and all that may be appropriate is help for the parent to cope with the sleeping pattern, rather than change it. Occasionally avoidance of dietary stimulants such as food additives and caffeine may make a difference. In the vast majority of cases however, what must be suggested is a change in the parents' responses, and a health visitor must exercise enormous tact if she is to help parents realise that they can alter the situation without making them feel that it has all been their fault in the first place.

Several excellent books on helping children to sleep well are available, (eg Douglas and Richman, 1984; Haslam, 1984), but often a parent will not turn to these until a problem has become established. By educating parents in appropriate ways of responding to their children during the night, and by using the handout, which can be given to parents before their babies reach the age at which they can 'waken at will', good sleeping patterns can often be established by the parents' efforts alone. This has two major benefits:

- By knowing how to avert problems, difficulties are less likely to occur, the parent is less dependent on professionals for advice, and self-esteem is enhanced.

- The methods advocated are based on the principle of responding to children in a consistent way and parents also learn to avoid unwittingly giving 'rewards' for undesirable behaviour. The skills thus learned are easily applied to other aspects of parenting and can be used to advantage in a variety of situations.

References

Douglas, J. and Richman, N. (1984) My Child Won't Sleep. Penguin, London.

Haslam, D. (1984) Sleepless Children. Futura, London.

Horne, J. (1981) Why we need to sleep. *New Scientist*, November, 429-431.

Newson, J. and Newson, E. (1965) Patterns of Infant Care in an Urban Community. Pelican, London.

Newson, J. and Newson, E. (1970) Four Years Old in an Urban Community. Pelican, London.

Seiler, E.R. (1968) Sleep Patterns in Children. *Practitioner*, **208**, 271-276.

Getting Your Baby to Sleep at Night

Some parents, either through good luck or good management, find that from the age of about three months their children sleep throughout the night, every night, settling happily at bedtime and waking full of energy in the morning. If this does not sound like your family, you are not alone – studies have shown that about *one third* of one-year-old babies have disrupted sleep patterns, and that means an awful lot of tired parents!

While there are certainly ways you might cope with regular night-time disturbances once they have become established, many parents feel that they could avoid a lot of stress if they were able to help their children develop acceptable sleep patterns while still babies. This handout shows how this might be done.

Sleep – what is it?

First, we have to know something of the nature of sleep. Sleep is essential to us all, but while some adults cope happily with five hours per night, most children require much more, and babies most of all. The 'average' baby of nine months might require about 14 hours' sleep out of 24; perhaps such a baby would sleep from 7.30pm to 6.30am, then have an hour's sleep in the morning and another nap in the afternoon.

If we look more closely at the sleep between 7.30pm and 6.30am we would see that she does not have the same depth of sleep throughout, but that in common with the rest of us, she alternates between very deep sleep, when she would be difficult to rouse, and periods of lighter sleep when at times she is almost awake, and indeed is certain to waken if disturbed. The speed with which she then goes back to sleep depends very much on how she has learnt to settle.

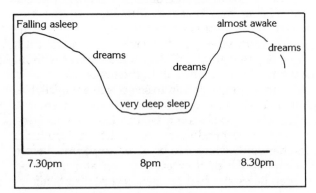

What happens when your baby falls asleep.
This kind of 'sleep cycle' will be repeated many times during the night.

Settling methods

Settling babies to sleep in the first few weeks of life becomes something of an endurance test for many parents. Most will adopt almost any method which works at the time, and this can include bottle or breast-feeding, giving a dummy, swaddling, rocking, patting, singing, encouraging thumb-sucking and taking for rides in the car.

While any of these methods may be ideal for very young babies, those of five or six months and older can very quickly become dependent on one method of settling to the exclusion of all others. The result of this is that not only is the rocking or feeding necessary at bedtime, but it becomes necessary several times a night during the baby's 'almost awake' period.

If the normal settling method is not then immediately available, the baby is aware that something is missing; she will not fall asleep without her required settling method because she does not know how to, and she is very likely to protest! An important factor begins to emerge here:

> If your baby requires your help for her preferred settling method, you will be disturbed every time she needs to get back to sleep.

Since she may be 'almost awake' seven or eight times a night, that can mean a lot of disturbance – so, what can you do?

The sucking connection

Little babies often like to suck until they are asleep, and will often fall asleep while feeding. If your baby is still doing this at six to seven months of age, it could be time to gently help your baby learn how to settle alone. This means regularly and consistently putting your baby in her cot at sleeping times *still awake*, but, does not necessarily mean that you must deprive her of breast or bottle, which can be offered equally well on awakening rather than on going to sleep. Alternatively, you can continue to give these at bedtime, providing that you do not let your baby fall asleep while still sucking.

It also does not mean that you will suffer a screaming baby for weeks on end because, with consistent behaviour on your part, your baby should learn her new routine well within a week. In this case, when your baby cries in her cot, at bedtime or during the night, you should go to her regularly to reassure her calmly, but *do not give the settling method* as a means of getting her to fall asleep. It is important that you do not offer any other settling method such as singing or rocking which requires your involvement in its place. You should find that after the first few nights your baby will quickly learn how to settle alone. She will continue to have several 'almost awake' spells every night, but will settle to sleep again if undisturbed, and will only cry persistently if in discomfort or pain.

The attention-seeker

Perhaps your baby is a little older and has proved herself capable of falling asleep without your assistance, but is beginning to show signs of wakefulness during the night. Sometimes you might feel that there is no reason for her to deliberately stay awake; you begin to get the feeling that she is 'playing you up'. From the baby's point of view, the explanation is simple:-

> It is much more fun to see mum or dad several times a night than to lie alone in a cot – even if they do get exceedingly cross!

The wakening habit can therefore become something of an attention-seeking routine, especially with babies of 10 months and more. When this results in repeated screaming for attention throughout the night, once again a consistent response on your part can pay dividends.

Be a bore!

Go to your baby when she cries, calmly tell her that it is time to go to sleep. Tuck her in if you wish, but keep verbal and physical contact to a minimum and leave the room quietly. Do not plead with her, sing to her, play with her, smack her or shout at her in an attempt to get some silence, as any of these responses can be more interesting (and rewarding) for your baby than going back to sleep. Simply repeat the above procedure every five or 10 minutes and remember your aim is to be as *boring as possible!*

The first and second night you try these tactics, you could find yourself getting out of bed up to 20 times, but for most parents the long-term benefits outweigh the short-term discomforts. By the fifth night you should see remarkable progress; unless your baby is most exceptionally determined, she will have realised that there is simply no point in making a fuss.

Can you help your baby to sleep well?

Try to:
- Establish a relaxed and predictable bedtime routine.
- Provide a comfortable sleeping environment.
- Put baby down for the night when sleepy but not overtired.
- Put baby in cot awake, both at bedtime and for daytime naps.
- Help baby learn to settle alone, without assistance (a baby with a dummy may require assistance if it keeps getting lost).
- Attend promptly to cries during the night but keep interaction brief; be as 'boring' as possible.
- Avoid giving any 'reward' for crying (eg singing, rocking) that your baby may wish you to repeat.
- Avoid leaving baby to cry for more than ten minutes at a time – give him the reassurance of a brief glimpse of you.
- Pick baby up in the morning and after daytime naps as promptly as you can and while he is still happy; avoid using cot or bedroom as a punishment.

10.30 am	Put in cot for morning nap. Cried for a few minutes then fell asleep till 11.15.
2.00pm	Fell asleep for 15 minutes while in pushchair.
7.30pm	Fell asleep while breastfeeding. Put in cot.
10.00pm	Cried. Husband went upstairs to rock to sleep (unsuccessfully) eventually brought baby down for breastfeed. Wide awake then, wanted to play.
11.30pm	Put in cot. Cried so much we picked him up again.
Midnight	Fell asleep in arms. Put in cot.
3.00am	Woke for breastfeed. Fell asleep in our bed and was left there until
5.00am	Woke again, fed for two minutes. Fell asleep. Put back in cot.
7.30am	Woke and cried. Took dummy and fell asleep for another hour.

Extract from a sleep diary kept by the mother of Robert, an eight month old boy. The boy could already settle alone – for his morning nap – so the mother began to put him down awake after early-evening and late-evening breastfeeds. She decided not to take baby into bed as she knew he would fall asleep feeding. Two weeks after this was written, Robert was sleeping regularly from 9.00pm to 7.00am.

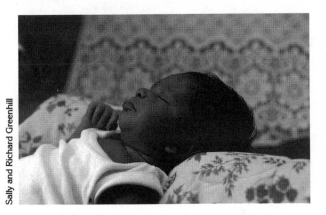

Sally and Richard Greenhill

Sleep diaries

Some parents keep a sleep diary as a means of identifying, preventing or solving sleeping problems. If you are attempting to correct sleep disruption it can be particularly useful to record your baby's night-time behaviour and your own responses towards her, before planning any change.

Time for change?

Many parents have found the ideas described in this handout work with just a little perseverance. If you think your baby's sleeping pattern should be changed, then choose a good time to start – not when you are especially tired or have visitors staying! Try to arrange to catch up on your own lost sleep by organising some alternative care for your baby for an hour or two on the first couple of days. Above all, do not struggle on alone – if you already have a sleeping problem in your family, whatever the age of the child, your health visitor should be able to provide the necessary advice and support, so that you too can enjoy some silent nights.

'Glue ear' is a common condition in childhood, and most parents are familiar with the term. The handout with this Patient Education Plus will help them understand the treatment offered.

Understanding 'glue ear'

Vanessa Martin, SRN, RSCN
Ward Sister, The Queen Elizabeth Hospital, King's Lynn, Norfolk

The insertion of a grommet for 'glue ear' remains the most frequent operation performed on children under general anaesthetic (Donaldson, 1987) so it is not surprising that the majority of parents and primary school children have heard of 'glue ear' and of grommets. Many do not really understand the condition, nor the function of a grommet, however because it is difficult in a busy outpatient clinic to explain adequately why we treat a nose or throat infection, or a nasal allergy when the child has been referred with a hearing problem. Parents ask why ear drops are not offered, why operations are delayed or why they vary from child to child. Many parents become confused, and this can lead to misunderstandings and lack of cooperation.

Diagnosis

Glue ear is a condition in which sterile fluid accumulates in the middle ear. The main clinical feature is a conductive deafness which may go unrecognised by the parents but be picked up on routine audiometry, which has been performed in schools since the 1950s, or by recognition of the presence of fluid in the middle ear by a general practitioner. In spite of intensive research in the last 15-20 years, the aetiology remains uncertain. What is known is that there is "eustachian tube dysfunction and defective ventilation of the middle ear", and the pathology of the middle ear mucosa shows a "hyperplasia of the mucous glands" (Cowan and Kerr, 1986).

Glue ear is not a new condition (Black, 1985a). Clear descriptions are documented from as early as 1860s, and there is some evidence of earlier recognition. Black (1985b) reports that there were many suggested causes, ranging from infant bottle feeding, lack of physical activity and poor hygiene to poor bowel habits and violent nose blowing. Today the most common theories are viral infections, allergy, unresolved acute otitis media, and adenoidal hypertrophy causing obstruction to the eustachian tube and consequently to the drainage. Eustachian malfunction causes glue ear in 90 per cent of children with cleft palate, claim Cowan and Kerr (1986), though other otologists may have different theories. This means that the medical treatment for this condition can vary tremendously.

Bibliography
Cotton, R.T. and Birman, C.W., Zalzal G.H. (1984) Serous otitis in children: medical and surgical aspects, diagnosis and management. *Clinical reviews in Allergy*, **2**, 329-43.
East, D.M. (1984) A layman's guide to grommets. *British Medical Journal*, **289**, 1596-98.
Shan, N. (1975) Glue ear – information for parents. Available from The Royal National Throat Nose and Ear Hospital, London.

Surgery

Children who fail to respond to medical treatment are offered surgery, which may include removal of the adenoids, a myringotomy (making a small radial incision into the tympanic membrane) and removal of the 'glue' by suction, and/or the insertion of a grommet. While adenoidectomy is a controversial form of therapy for treating glue ear, insertion of a grommet is generally agreed to have benefits (Donaldson, 1987). Ideally, it is inserted for as long as the eustachian tube fails to function, as its aim is to temporarily replace it, but this period is difficult to predict.

References

Black, N. (1985a) Glue ear: The new dyslexia? *British Medical Journal,* **290,** 1963-65.

Black, N. (1985b) Causes of glue ear: An historical review of theories and evidence. *Journal of Laryngology and Otology,* **99,** 953-66.

Donaldson, J.D. (1987) Otitis media update *Journal of Otolaryngology,* **16,** 221-23.

Marks, N.J. and Mills, R.P. (1983) Swimming and grommets. *Journal of the Royal Society of Medicine,* **76,** 23-26.

Cowan, D.C. and Kerr, A.I.G., (1986) Paediatric otolaryngology – Secretory Otitis Media, 145-48.

Smelt, G.J.C. and Yeoh, L.H., (1984) Swimming and grommets. *Journal of Laryngology and Otology,* **98,** 243-45.

Stangerup, S.E. and Tos M. (1986) Treatment of secretory otitis and pneumatisation. *Laryngoscopy,* **96,** 680-84.

Controversy

Acknowledgments

I would like to thank B.P. Cvijetic, FRCS, and N.P. Chowdary DLO, for their help and advice, Norma Spooner for her practical and secretarial help, Ann Osborne for finding relevant articles, and Sarah Oldfield for typing this manuscript.

Insertion of a grommet maintains hearing, ventilates the middle ear, leads to the recovery of the middle ear mucosa and, according to Stangerup and Tos (1986), has a positive effect on the process of pneumatisation. Their survey suggested that children with glue ear who are treated with grommets develop a significantly larger mastoid cell system. On the other hand, Black (1985a) states that "the use of tympanostomy tubes may possibly cause long term harm. In one study nearly half the children who had tubes inserted were found to have tympanosclerosis of the ear drum in the year or two after operation". Surgical treatment remains controversial.

As the above description illustrates, glue ear is a highly complex condition. The handout overleaf is designed to outline the disease and possible treatments in a simple and concise form, free from complicated medical terms, although it cannot answer every question parents might ask. It can be photocopied and distributed freely to parents at the time that surgery is suggested.

Even with the declared intention of simplicity, we can not avoid controversy. The care of a grommet is also debated by otologists. It seems to be widely accepted that swimming is allowed. The hole in the grommet is small enough to keep water out, and Smelt and Yeoh (1984) say that children with grommets inserted are no more likely to develop otorrhoea if they do swim than if they do not. Whether children's ears should be protected during hair washing is uncertain. Marks and Mills. (1983) say that soaps and detergents, by lowering the surface tension, make water more likely to enter the middle ear. Protection of the ear for hair washing is included in the handout even though some otologists may feel this unnecessary.

Understanding 'Glue Ear'

In a normal ear, sound waves pass down the ear canal and through to the inner ear by vibrating the ear drum and ossicles, which are small bones in the middle ear. The inner ear then transmits those sounds to the brain.

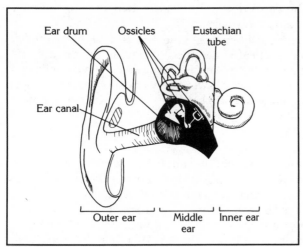

A normal ear

In glue ear, the sound waves can not pass through the middle ear because of a sticky glue-like fluid which prevents the ear drum and the ossicles from vibrating.

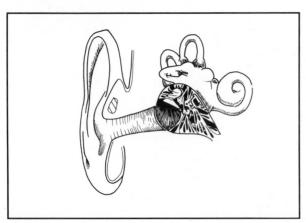

Glue ear

Why does this happen?
The eustachian tube, which runs from the middle ear to the back of the nose, opens on swallowing and allows air to enter the middle ear. Glue develops because the eustachian tube is not functioning properly.

Causes
The causes of poor function of the eustachian tube are not always clear. Repeated infections, enlarged adenoids, allergies or weakness of the muscles in the area of the eustachian tube can all contribute.

Treatment
The following may be tried:
- Antibiotics to clear infections.
- Decongestants to unblock nasal passages.
- Removal of adenoids, which lie at the back of

the nose near the openings of the eustachian tubes.
- A myringotomy – making of a small hole in the ear drum and removal of the 'glue' by suction.
- The insertion of a grommet into the ear drum.

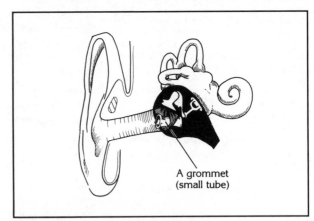

A grommet (small tube)

The purpose of a grommet
A grommet temporarily takes over the function of the eustachian tube. It allows air to enter the middle ear and gives the ear the opportunity to recover. Different grommets are selected to stay in place for different lengths of time. Some come out on their own after a few months, some remain for longer, and others have to be surgically removed.

If a short-term grommet has been inserted but the 'glue' collects again, it may be necessary to insert another type of grommet.

Looking after a grommet
(1) When washing your child's hair, it is preferable if you place a piece of cotton wool smeared with vaseline into your child's ear hole (entrance of the ear canal.) This is because soapy water can irritate the ear.
(2) Your child may swim, but do not allow him to swim under water, or dive.
(3) If your child should develop a discharge from his ear, or severe pain, contact your GP.
(4) You will be asked to attend the out patient department for a follow up. The surgeon will check whether the grommet is functioning and with the aid of a hearing test, will check that your child continues to hear normally.

Glue ear that is not treated
The condition of 'glue ear' is likely to improve in your child from the age of seven to eight years onwards. However, if persistent 'glue ear' is not treated before this time:
- The child may be slower to learn and to develop because he is not hearing properly.
- Changes may occur in the ear drum and the middle ear resulting in permanent deafness.

Useful contacts
Ward ....
Phone ....
Ward sister/Charge nurse ....

It is now rare for women to have the opportunity to learn about breastfeeding from friends and relatives, so advice from midwives, health visitors and other nurses can be of considerable importance in helping new mothers to establish and maintain successful breastfeeding.

Successful breastfeeding

Chloe Fisher, MTD
Senior Midwife, Community, Central Oxfordshire

Helen Minns, MTD
Midwifery Tutor, John Radcliffe Hospital, Oxford

Breastfeeding has been the subject of considerable emotive debate over the last four decades because, during this time, social and attitudinal changes have enabled women to choose whether or not to breastfeed. The advantages of successful breastfeeding for the baby's health and for the relationship between the mother and the baby are well documented (see, for example, Ebrahim, 1978) (Table 1) and problems which may be experienced should be understood by the mother so that she can, if possible, overcome them. For those mothers who decide that the disadvantages to them of breastfeeding (Table 2) outweigh the advantages to the baby, and for the very small number of mothers who are unable to breastfeed, appropriate information and advice about alternative feeding should be given. Midwives can have an influential role in building and maintaining the confidence of some mothers, enabling them to start and to continue with breastfeeding where otherwise they may be deterred by the problems they encounter, or by social pressures.

Essential requirements for successful breastfeeding

That the woman wishes to breastfeed Most women choose to breastfeed simply because they want to. They have nurtured their baby thoughout pregnancy and it seems natural to continue to do so after birth. Women who wish to breastfeed will be anxious to do as much as possible during pregnancy to prepare themselves, but there is no evidence to support the value of any physical preparation of the breast (Hytten, 1958). Changes occur naturally during pregnancy, including the development of the Montgomery's tubercules (the little glands in the areola which produce a lubricant for the skin), increased areolar pigmentation and the formation of colostrum, which starts early in pregnancy. Successful breastfeeding does not depend on the mother's skin colour or the shape or size of the breasts or nipples.

- Food exactly matches the baby's nutritional requirements and changes with the baby's needs.
- A ready supply of clean food, at body temperature, is available wherever the mother is and without any special preparation.
- Colostrum, the major constituent of the feed during the first few days after birth, contains a rich mixture of antibodies which confer passive immunity to the baby.
- The close relationship between mother and baby is facilitated and improved by breastfeeding.
- The majority of mothers find that breastfeeding is a most satisfying activity.

Table 1. Advantages of breastfeeding.

- Mothers may encounter social antagonism toward breastfeeding and may feel restricted in their freedom to breastfeed and to maintain social contacts.

- Mothers may experience some of the painful and distressing problems which result from poor positioning of the baby at the breast.

- Mothers may experience leaking breasts and this may be inconvenient, but the problem usually improves with time.

Table 2. Present disadvantages of breastfeeding.

No artificial restrictions on length or frequency of feeds A few babies appear eager to start breastfeeding almost as soon as they are born while others may not show any interest for some time. Probably the most important factor is to be able to help the baby to feed as soon as it is ready. There is no advantage to the mother, or her baby, in restricting the duration of early feeds. Research has shown that unrestricted feeding reduces the incidence of sore nipples and encourages earlier and more generous milk production (Illingworth, 1952 and Salariya, Easton and Cater, 1978). The most common feeding pattern in the first two days is of fairly long feeds with long intervals between, but soon the baby will require more frequent feeds. The volume and rate of milk transfer varies with each mother and baby (Woolridge, Baum and Drewett, 1982).

Correctly positioning the baby at the breast The baby has to latch on to its mother's breast by drawing the nipple and areola into its mouth (Figure 1). To achieve this the mother must elicit the rooting reflex by touching the baby's mouth to the nipple so that it opens wide and the tongue goes down and forward. She must then quickly move the baby towards the breast so that the bottom lip makes contact well away from the base of the nipple (Fisher, 1981). This will enable the baby to draw the glandular tissue behind the areola, containing the lactiferous ducts, into its mouth (Table 3).

The handout can be photocopied for distribution to parents.

References

Ardran, G.M., Kemp, F.H. and Lind, J.A. (1958) Cineradiographic study of breastfeeding. *British Journal of Radiology,* **31,** 156-62.

Ebrahim, G.J. (1978) Breastfeeding: the biological option. The Macmillan Press Ltd, London and Basingstoke.

Fisher, C. (1981) Breastfeeding — a midwife's view. *Journal of Maternity and Child Health,* **6,** 2, 52-57.

Hytten, F.E. (1958) The development of the nipple during pregnancy. *The Lancet,* **i,** 1201-04.

Illingworth, R.S. and Stone, D.G. (1952) Self demand feeding in a maternity unit. *The Lancet,* **i,** 683.

Salariya, E.M., Easton, P.M. and Cates, J.I. (1978) Duration of breastfeeding after early initiation and frequent feeding. *The Lancet,* **ii,** 1141.

Woolridge, M.W., Baum, J.D. and Drewett, R.F. (1982) Individual patterns of milk intake during breastfeeding. *Early Human Development,* **7,** 3, 265-72.

Bibliography

Health Education Authority (1989) From Birth to Five Years.
This is an excellent guide for parents and parents-to-be on all aspects of pregnancy, childbirth and early child care. It is available free of charge from the Health Education Authority.

- Breastfeeding does not cause pain.

- The nipple is not damaged.

- Efficient milk transfer occurs, helping the baby to obtain its calorie requirement from the high fat hindmilk (Hytten, 1954).

- The baby will come off the breast spontaneously and feeds will not be prolonged.

- Engorgement is prevented.

- The breast does not have to be held away from the baby's nose.

- The baby will not be restless while feeding.

- The baby may at times be satisfied with one breast only or may require only a little on the second side.

- Problems with wind and colic will be reduced.

- The baby's growth and development will proceed satisfactorily.

Table 3. Benefits of correct positioning.

Figure 1. Correct positioning of the baby ensures proper feeding without damage to the nipple.

Breastfeeding

How babies feed
The baby takes a mouthful of breast with the nipple and so draws into its mouth the breast tissue where the milk pools during breastfeeding. The baby obtains the milk by stripping it from the breast with its tongue and only uses suction to stay attached to the breast. The composition of the milk changes throughout the feed: the proportion of fat, important for the baby's growth, increases continuously.

After birth
When the baby is ready to feed it should be 'teased' (Figure 1) by being moved gently against the breast until it opens its mouth wide. When this happens, its tongue moves down and forwards. Aiming the bottom lip about half an inch away from the base of the nipple, move the baby quickly to the breast. Do not try to put the breast into the baby's mouth as this distorts the shape. The correct position (Figure 2) is most easily achieved if you lean slightly forward. In the early days it may be more comfortable to feed lying on your side; you will probably need help to position the baby. Never be afraid to ask your midwife for help and advice on correct positioning of the baby: this is essential for successful breastfeeding.

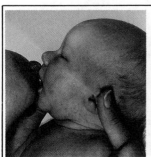 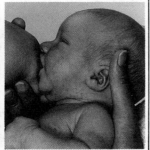

Figure 1. 'Tease' the baby.   *Figure 2. The correct position.*

Timing of the first feed
The first feed of the baby initiates lactation and although many people believe that it is important to feed the baby as soon as possible after birth, it is probably more important to feed the baby when he or she is first ready, sometime during the first 24 hours. Allow the baby to feed for as long as required on the first breast. He or she will let go spontaneously. This is now an opportunity to change the baby's nappy and then to offer the second breast. Some babies only want one breast at each feed. The common pattern in the first two days is of fairly long feeds with long intervals between, but babies soon want to feed more frequently. By the end of the first week many babies settle down to an average of six feeds in 24 hours but with some variation in the times between, and the breasts will have become much softer.

Some breastfeeding problems
Sore or cracked nipples. For many years it was thought that limiting the length of early feeds would prevent sore nipples. This was wrong, and actually increased the incidence of early problems, which occur when the baby is incorrectly positioned.
Engorged breasts. Engorgement is another problem that may occur in the early days. It is caused by limiting the duration of early feeds or as a result of poor milk extraction due to poor positioning. If your baby is allowed to feed well, your breasts will soon improve. If nipples become flattened, and it is difficult to feed, ask your midwife for help.

Lumpy and inflamed breasts
If your breasts become lumpy or inflamed (mastitis), this indicates that the baby isn't feeding correctly and milk is building up in one or more segment of the breast. The problem will normally improve if the baby is allowed to feed well from the first breast and takes only a little or no milk from the second side. This feeding strategy is much better than offering the baby both breasts equally at each feed. You should consult your doctor if the problem persists as infection may occur.

Food and drink
Most breastfeeding mothers have a good appetite and yet do not gain weight. It is not necessary to increase calorie intake in order to breastfeed successfully. Milk is not essential in your diet, although it is an excellent, well-balanced food. There are no foods to be avoided unless, as sometimes happens, the baby becomes fussy in response to something in the mother's diet. You will drink more in response to the natural increase in thirst that occurs in lactating women. An artificial increase in fluid intake will have no effect on the volume of milk you produce.

If any problems do arise, not at all uncommon in the first few days, it is essential to seek help.

―――――――――――――― **Useful addresses** ――――――――――――――

Alexandra House, Oldham Terrace, London W3 6NH. Telephone 01-992 8637.

Local branches run antenatal classes. Also give breastfeeding advice and practical postnatal help. Write or phone for information.

BM 3424, London WC1 3XX. Telephone 01-404 5011.

Offers help and information to women who want to breastfeed their babies. Counsellors answer mothers' questions by phone. Local groups hold discussions on breastfeeding, birth and parenthood. Send a stamped addressed envelope for details.

10, Herschel Road, London SE23. Telephone 01-778 4769.

Offers a 24-hour telephone service to breastfeeding mothers. Runs local support groups.

Weaning can be a stressful time for parents of young babies. Much emotional importance is put on feeding, and minor problems can easily be blown out of proportion by worried parents.

A parent's guide to weaning

Elizabeth M. Horne, MA
Editorial Director, The Professional Nurse

Myra Ibbotson, PhD, BSc, SRD
Freelance Dietitian

Weaning is the gradual transition made by babies from a diet comprised largely of milk, to a more diverse diet consisting predominantly of solid foods. The cultural and social background of different families lead to different expectations and beliefs about weaning on the part of the child's parents, and can lead to controversy over the ideal timing and planning of the weaning process. Nurses and health visitors can do much to help parents make the weaning process as stress free as possible for both the parents and child by giving appropriate advice and allaying unnecessary worries.

Psychological aspects

The intake of a good balance of different nutrients in the form of foods and fluids is essential for normal growth and development during childhood and for health throughout our lives. Perhaps because it is such a basic requirement for life, feeding is a powerfully emotive activity, and, for parents, one which may cause most anxiety if problems arise along the route toward a healthy 'normal' diet. Parents – and particularly mothers who are breastfeeding – see the weaning process as representing and illustrating the changes in the relationship between the adult and the growing child, from complete dependence as a newborn baby to the relative independence of the child (Lowen, 1980).

The associations small children attach to new foods and flavours may strongly influence their food preferences later in life and the new foods encountered during the weaning process set important precedents for the future.

The levels of confidence and competence with which a mother approaches the feeding of her baby can be extensively supported or badly undermined by the advice and feedback she gets when the baby is routinely checked and weighed. *Absolute* weight gain, against one of the standard growth charts, is not as important as a pattern of steady weight gain and a clearly healthy baby, even if the baby weighs less for its age than the average. Babies (and adults) vary considerably in the body weight which is 'normal' for them. If parents are made to feel they are underfeeding the baby, their concern and loss of confidence can actually lead to feeding problems as mealtimes become emotionally charged events instead of what is ideally a fairly uneventful part of the normal routine.

Parents may seek advice and help from GPs and health visitors, particularly if problems are encountered. The handout on pages 67 to 69 may be helpful to parents and can be photocopied for distribution or adapted freely.

Reference
Lowen, A. (1980) Fear of Life. Macmillan Publishing Company, New York.

Weaning Your Baby

Weaning is the gradual transition made by babies from a diet comprised largely of milk to a more diverse diet consisting predominantly of solids.

When should weaning start?

There are no strict rules, and as with so many developments, children vary considerably in their requirements and the speed at which these change. However, unless there are special medical reasons, no baby should start being offered solid foods before the age of four months, and most babies will certainly need solid foods by the time they reach 12 lbs (5.5 kg) in weight. You need to introduce your baby to the new tastes of solid foods ahead of his or her actual need for these foods. Even for a very small baby, whose weight will not reach 12 lbs for several weeks, you should start introducing tiny tastes when he or she is seven or eight months old. If you leave it much later, your child will find the new tastes and feeding methods less easy to accept.

First solid foods

Start by feeding very tiny quantities (1-2 teaspoons) of solid foods at each feed and the usual amount of milk. At first, use baby rice or other gluten free cereals and after a fortnight or so start to offer a variety of flavours. Never force him or her to take

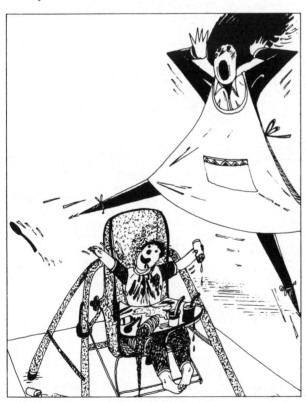

any – it is important to respect the definite preferences your baby will show. 'Solid' foods should be semi-liquid in texture: lumps or pips may make your baby choke if swallowed.

At first, solid foods are needed only for the extra calories they provide. Your baby will be getting enough of all the other nutrients – proteins, fats,

vitamins and minerals – from milk. *Any bland food*, so long as it is liquidised or mashed, will provide this: potato or carrots mashed with milk or gravy or stewed and puréed fruit (avoid those with pips, such as gooseberries) would be ideal. Baby rice and other gluten-free cereals are often chosen as the first solid foods and are rich in iron. Don't add salt, which adds a strain to the baby's kidneys, and avoid spices which may burn the baby's mouth or irritate the digestive system. Too much fat or sugar will also upset digestion.

Commercially available cans and jars of baby food provide too great a quanity to be really useful at this stage – your baby will only need one or two teaspoons of food at each feed and, once opened, jars and cans will only remain fresh for 24 hours, even in the fridge. Don't feed from the jar as saliva will spoil the food. Transfer a little into a bowl first. Dehydrated foods are more useful because they can be used gradually.

It will take a little time for your baby to learn to take food from a spoon instead of sucking, and it is best not to try offering food on a spoon when your baby is very hungry and keen to suck. Offer a teaspoonful of solid food part way through a feed of milk. Use a small spoon and hold this just between his or her lips so that your baby can suck the food far enough back in the mouth to swallow.

Solids as meals

Gradually your baby will show that he or she wants more solid food, and may want to start a meal with solids, or refuse more milk after solids have been eaten. Enthusiasm for solid food may vary from day to day but let the baby take the lead: don't try and force the pace. Food should be fun! Let your baby play with his or her food and spoons, this is how they learn to handle food for themselves. Equip your baby, yourself and the floor to expect the mess which will result!

'Finger foods', such as a raw carrot, crust or rusk, are useful snacks and will help your baby to learn more about feeding him or herself. Your baby will only be able to move food from the front to the back of the mouth when he or she is about five months old.

The weaning process

An important element of your baby's early feeding is the comfort he or she derives from sucking. During weaning, the amount of sucking will decrease and your baby's new skills of feeding from a spoon and drinking from a cup will increase. A teacher-beaker with a lid and spout will help your baby learn to drink from a cup, but the comfort of sucking will still be needed – especially at bedtime, and perhaps at the first feed in the morning. Most children will give this up naturally at about the time of their first birthday. If you are breastfeeding, but reluctant to continue for this long, it may be necessary to introduce a bottle for milk at bedtime.

How much food?

A six month old baby needs, on average, about 800 calories per day, and will be getting most of this from milk, which also provides all the protein, fats, minerals and vitamins required.

As your baby's milk consumption drops, plan foods which provide calories, iron and vitamins A, D and C. He or she will still be getting enough protein, calcium and B group vitamins by drinking a pint of milk a day. This can be included in the preparation of other foods, such as scrambled egg, cereals or custard. Commercially available 'high protein' foods will have no extra benefit; nor will meat or fish.

Which foods?

As long as you avoid added salt, hot spices, alcohol, coffee and tea, there is little which adults would normally eat which the baby should not have, but food must be semi-liquid and presented in tiny amounts. The ready-prepared baby cereals are valuable foods fortified with iron and vitamins and convenient to use.

Cans or jars of baby food tend to provide less concentrated nutrients than the equivalent home-cooked versions, but are much more convenient to use. You will probably want to use both options.

If you are worried

Worrying about the amount of food your baby eats will destroy the trust you need to develop with your baby, and will increase the likelihood of problems. If your baby's weight is increasing steadily, and he or she is taking at least milk and is active and lively, there is probably no need for worry. Contact your health visitor or GP if you *are* worried, or want to discuss developments in your baby's feeding patterns.

	Home-prepared foods	Commercially-prepared foods
Convenience for you	Can be a nuisance to prepare for the baby alone, although are no trouble if you are cooking for others and can adapt the meal. Awkward to carry hygienically or to find in strange places.	Are never any trouble to prepare. Easy to carry with you and serve anywhere.
Food value	Variable. Freshly cooked and quickly served food will be excellent; leftovers will not be good for her.	Always excellent and always the same, although different varieties have unexpected differences in calorie value, etc. Until recently these contained added sugar, which should be avoided.
Adaptability	Can be adapted to suit your baby's individual appetite, taste and digestion. Can also be served in different ways to make a change in appearance or texture. Different kinds of food can be served separately so that the baby can discover what foods she does and does not like and choose what to eat and what to leave. Familiar foods can be made suitable for finger-feeding as she gets older, with cubed or grated, rather than puréed, vegetables, cheeses, etc.	Cannot be adapted at all. A meal is a meal, with everything mixed together so that a fat baby must have all the carbohydrate if she is to have the meat; a bored baby must see a dish that always looks the same, and a baby cannot separate the taste of peas from carrots. Finger-feeding is impossible. "Lumpy" varieties made for older babies are often disliked.
Preparation for family meals	Excellent; she will become accustomed to various tastes and textures and eventually see that she is eating the same as you.	Not good. All tend to be bland, so that "apple variety" is no preparation for the tartness of fresh stewed apple. She may become so used to consistently smooth textures that she dislikes food that needs chewing. Her food does not even look like yours.

Table 1. Home prepared and commercially prepared foods compared.
(Reproduced with kind permission from Baby and Child, by Penelope Leach, Dorling Kindersley, London, 1977.)

The Weaning Process

Stage 1
eg 4 months*

Early morning:
Breast or bottle feed.

Breakfast:
Try one or two teaspoons of baby rice as well as the breast or bottle feed.

Lunch:
Breast or bottle feed.

Tea:
Breast or bottle feed.

Evening:
Breast or bottle feed.

Stage 2
4½ months

Early morning:
Breast or bottle feed.

Breakfast:
One or two teaspoons of baby rice then breast or bottle feed.

Lunch:
Try one or two teaspoons of sieved vegetables or strained broth. Then breast or bottle feed.

Tea:
Breast or bottle feed.

Evening:
Breast or bottle feed.

Stage 3
4¾ months

Early morning:
Breast or bottle feed.

Breakfast:
One or two teaspoons of baby rice then breast or bottle feed.

Lunch:
Try puréed meat or fish with sieved vegetables. Then breast or bottle feed.

Tea:
Try a little fruit purée as well as the breast or bottle feed.

Evening:
Breast or bottle feed.

Stage 4
5-6 months

Early morning:
Breast or bottle feed.

Breakfast:
Still give baby rice, but try a few teaspoons of lightly boiled egg yolk too. Then breast or bottle feed.

Lunch:
Puréed meat or fish with sieved vegetables. Then a little stewed fruit. Try giving a drink of water or well diluted fruit juice instead of the feed.

Tea:
Try a mashed banana or other soft fruit as well as the breast or bottle feed.

Evening:
Breast or bottle feed if your baby is still hungry.

Stage 5
6-7 months

Early morning:
Breast or bottle feed, if still needed.

Breakfast:
Try cereal or porridge and lightly scrambled egg. Try giving a drink of milk instead of the breast or bottle feed. Ask your health visitor whether the milk should be boiled first.
Remember, as soon as your baby starts on household milk, it's important to give vitamin drops. Ask your health visitor for advice.

Lunch:
Try giving minced or mashed food instead of puréed food. Give meat or fish with vegetables. Then try ground rice or semolina, egg custard or jelly. Give a drink of water or well diluted fruit juice.

Tea:
Try a cheese or other savoury sandwich. Then fruit or yogurt. Try giving a drink of milk instead of the feed.

Stage 6
7-8 months

Early morning:
Try giving a drink of water or fruit juice.

Breakfast:
Still give cereal and then boiled egg with wholemeal toast and butter. Give a drink of milk.

Lunch:
Try cheese or fish, or minced meat, chicken or liver, with mashed vegetables. Then milk pudding or stewed fruit and a drink of water or fruit juice.

Tea:
Bread and butter with savoury spread or cottage cheese. Then fruit or yogurt and a drink of milk.

Stage 7
9-12 months

Early morning:
Drink of water or fruit juice.

Breakfast:
Cereal then bacon, egg or fish with toast and butter and a drink of milk.

Lunch:
Try giving chopped food instead of minced or mashed food. Give meat, fish or cheese. Then milk pudding, fruit or egg custard with a drink of water or fruit juice.

Tea:
Fish, meat or cheese sandwiches with a drink of milk.

*Remember: the age babies need to start solid food varies. Your baby may start earlier or later than four months and you should adjust the chart accordingly.

Febrile convulsions occur in children under the age of five. Although they are unlikely to cause lasting damage, they can cause great anxiety for parents. Nurses can help to alleviate this anxiety by giving parents effective education about the condition.

What are febrile convulsions?

Lorenzo C. Visentin
Third Year Student Nurse, New Cross Hospital, Wolverhampton

A child can produce a high temperature with a very minor illness, so it is not surprising that febrile convulsions occur in approximately 2.5 per cent of all children. Febrile or infantile convulsions are seizures that occur in the context of a febrile illness in a previously normal child (Brunner and Suddarth, 1986).

Febrile convulsions, as distinct from other seizure disorders (epilepsy, focal seizures and myoclonic fits), always accompany intercurrent infection such as pharyngitis, tonsilitis and otitis, and often simply coryza. The child presents with a core temperature of at least 38.8°C and an average age of 18 months, although these convulsions can occur at any time between six months and three years. It is rare to see febrile convulsions in a child over five.

As with all paediatric disorders, the convulsions cause the parents great anxiety. It is therefore essential that nurses offer and reinforce reassuring information to prevent undue anxiety, direct confrontation, in naturally concerned parents. Such anxiety can, in extreme cases, result in direct confrontation between parents and nurse.

Adverse events

Adverse events are harmful for children when they arouse more anxiety than the child can cope with. If a parent is anxious and tearful about the child being in hospital, this anxiety may be conveyed to the child and increase his or her distress (Davies, 1984). This makes parental education essential. The handout on page 559 is a simple, comprehensive guide to febrile convulsions intended for parents of children admitted to a paediatric unit. The information it includes gives the parents the opportunity to mentally rehearse a stressful event, so when it actually takes place there should be less emotional disturbance. A parent prepared for any care given to their child, either in or out of hospital, needs to feel in control of the situation. This feeling can be passed subconsciously through to the child, so the child then feels less distressed.

Parents of children admitted to hospital for febrile convulsions need help, understanding and reassurance – to them, their child is of paramount importance. As the convulsions occur only in the context of a febrile illness, the onset is likely to have been sudden with no predisposing factors other than a runny nose, so the parents are likely to be shocked by them. The first piece of reassurance anxious parents should receive is a warm welcome, while the child's safety is attended to.

Nursing action

Immediate nursing action involves reducing the child's temperature and preserving a patent airway. The child should not be restrained, and the convulsion's type should be accurately recorded, including its duration and severity. It is also important to give the parents an opportunity to become involved in their child's care. There must be a constructive discussion between the nurse and parents to establish what each expects of the other, where the gaps are and whose expertise fills them. If this is not done, it may be presumed that one or other is responsible for an aspect of the child's care and the gap is filled with frustration and dissatisfaction on both sides (Brewis, 1986).

It must be remembered that a common explanation for fever is misinterpretation of normal temperature reading (Brunner and Suddarth, 1986). Routine observation of temperature gives an ideal opportunity to teach parents the correct technique and how to analyse thermometer readings. Normal temperature ranges in children are:

- Oral   36.4 – 37.4°C
- Rectal   36.2 – 37.8°C
- Axillary   35.9 – 36.7°C

Parental guidance

Parents are likely to be the primary carers when the child is discharged home (Williams, 1987), so it is essential they are given a simple yet comprehensive guide to febrile convulsions; the recurrence rate is quite high – 40-50 per cent for a second convulsion and 15 per cent for a third. Verbal emphasis is needed as well as the written guide, especially when attempting to dispel old wives' tales such as sweating out a fever. Going through each stage of the guide with the parents gives them the opportunity to assimilate all the information they are receiving and to ask appropriate questions. Although time-consuming, the verbal reiteration of the information contained in the guide may be vital – parents do not necessarily have good reading ability, and those with a poor reading ability should be taken into consideration (Williams, 1987).

Once the child's condition has stabilised, teaching the parents simple first aid procedures such as the recovery position is useful. This easily learnt technique may appear complicated at first, but it is simple and may be life-saving. It is important to emphasise the need for non-restraint, to ensure parents are aware that they may unintentionally harm their child if they attempt restraint during a convulsion. When demonstrating how to maintain a patent airway, it is also important to tell parents not to force anything between the child's teeth. (Children occasionally bite their tongues at the onset of a convulsion, but will not damage it any further once the fit has started).

Recurrence

The high recurrence rate of febrile convulsions is influenced by a number of factors. The child's age is important, as the risk of recurrence is greater in younger children. There appears to be a familial tendency to convulsions, and those with a positive family history are more susceptible to recurring convulsions. Thirty per cent of recurrences occur within the first six months after the first seizure, and all recurrences (about 40-50 per cent of all cases) occur within 30 months. Girls are more likely than boys to have a recurrent febrile convulsion. Interestingly the risk of developing non-febrile convulsions is low (approximately 3 per cent) – children at risk are those with persistently abnormal electroencephalograms, central nervous system infections, prolonged febrile seizures (ie, above 20-30 minutes) and those who experience multiple febrile convulsions during one 24 hour period. Children who have this increased risk should be assessed and further guidance offered. Information leaflets are a cheap aid which can provide useful guidance and advice when properly explained (Williams, 1987), but they should never replace the specialised advice offered by paediatric nurses on a one-to-one basis with parents.

The handout overleaf can be photocopied or adapted for use with parents.

References

Brewis, E. (1986) Parental prerogatives. *Nursing Times*, **82**, 51,34-35.

Brunner, L.S. and Suddarth, D.S. (1986) The Lippincott Manual of Paediatric Nursing. Harper and Row, London.

Davies, C. (1984) Mother's anxiety may increase child's distress. *Nursing Mirror*, **158**, 18,30-31

Williams, J. (1987) Home nursing for parents. *Nursing Times*, **83**, 19,53-54.

If your child has suffered a febrile convulsion . . .

Your child has suffered a fit with a high temperature – a febrile convulsion. This is always caused by an infection like a cough or a cold, and there is a chance that another convulsion may occur (although this only happens in half of all cases), but if you follow a few simple rules another convulsion may be avoided. This handout will help you both to avoid your child having another convulsion and to know what to do if this should happen.

So if your child develops a cold or sore throat or can't hear properly (an ear infection) or simply has a cough and a runny nose:

Do's

Do take your child's temperature – leave the thermometer under the armpit for a full minute. Normal temperature varies slightly according to such things as the time of day, but it should fall between 36.5 and 37.5°C. If temperature is higher:

Do take off most of your child's clothes and open windows. This will cool the room and your child tremendously.

Do stay with the child – remember he or she may feel poorly and need comfort – also watch those open windows – accidents can still happen.

Do give a paracetamol syrup (such as Calpol) from the chemist, following the instructions on the bottle for the dose.

Do give plenty of drinks – with a little sugar added, as your child will be losing a lot of fluid by sweating, which must be replaced.

Do phone the family doctor, who will be pleased to see your child and may arrange hospital admission if necessary.

Do phone the children's ward. We will be happy to help and there is always a trained specialist nurse on the ward available for advice.

Don'ts

Don't insist on your child staying in bed. Children with a temperature don't always feel poorly and the bedclothes don't help bring down their temperature.

Don't listen to old wives' tales such as sweating out a fever – this is positively dangerous.

Don't hesitate to bring your child to casualty or direct to the children's ward.

Don't sponge your child with cold water, this will make the temperature fall too rapidly.

If your child has another fit

Remember, if your child does have another fit, that children almost always come out of it themselves – even if they go blue for a short time. There are a few things you can do to ensure safety:

1. Clear the area around the child to prevent any accidents.

2. Turn the child onto his or her side, into the recovery position.

3. Do not put anything into the child's mouth. Once the fit has started children do not bite their tongues.

4. Stay with your child but do not attempt to restrain him or her.

5. Dial 999 and ask for an ambulance.

For the future

It is extremely unlikely that your child will have suffered any permanent damage, but there is a chance that there may be a recurrence. By the time he or she goes to school, the chance of another fit will have all but disappeared. Do learn more about First Aid from one of the voluntary organisations such as St Johns Ambulance Brigade, the British Red Cross or St Andrew's Ambulance Association (Scotland). Their number will be in the phone book.

Finally remember if you are ever in any doubt, always ask and find out!

Useful phone numbers

Doctor . . . .

Children's Ward . . . .

Health visitor . . . .

Diabetes

If patients with diabetes are to monitor their blood glucose effectively it is important that they are given all the necessary information about diabetes and that they are sufficiently motivated to carry out their tests regularly. Nurses play an important part in teaching and assessing suitability for the method.

Blood glucose monitoring:
Teaching effective techniques

Sheila Reading, MSc, BSc, SRN
Diabetes Research Sister, Southampton University

Successful diabetic management involves patients taking responsibility for their own care. Blood glucose monitoring is a relatively easy, accurate and convenient tool, enabling those who have been educated about diabetes and the measuring and meaning of test results to improve their control and achieve normal blood glucose levels.

Teaching and support

The nurse plays an important role in both teaching good blood glucose monitoring techniques and also in supporting patients, helping them maintain and use this new skill to achieve good diabetic control on a long-term basis. It is important to help patients accept and actively take responsibility for their own care. This will involve providing them with all the essential information about their type of diabetes, the implications of this for their own monitoring and the use they can then make of these readings. Patients must decide which form of monitoring to adopt, and therefore need information, advice and support in deciding between blood and urine glucose monitoring.

Effective patient teaching depends on first assessing the patient's knowledge of diabetes and level of motivation to achieve good blood glucose control. Individuals will, of course, vary in their initial level of knowledge, and the amount of detail they will want and be able to effectively assimilate and use. The nurse's approach and choice of teaching aids (handouts, diagrams and so on) should therefore take this into account.

Assess patients' understanding

Nurses must also assess the effectiveness of their teaching: one approach to this is to ask patients to explain or to demonstrate their monitoring techniques. The handout opposite may be helpful in teaching blood glucose monitoring techniques, and can be photocopied for distribution to clients.

The patients' level of motivation is very important: unless they are motivated and accept the need for good control they will probably gain only a poor understanding of the significance and use of test results, and will derive little benefit from self monitoring.

Monitoring Blood Glucose at Home

You need to monitor the level of glucose in your blood daily or several times each day, so that you know how effectively you are keeping control of this. Blood glucose should be as close to normal as possible; this normal level can vary between 2.6 and 6.6 mmols/litre.

You will probably have discussed the advantages and disadvantages of both blood and urine glucose monitoring with your diabetic liaison nurse or health visitor. Blood glucose monitoring is much more informative than urine testing.

Benefits of blood glucose monitoring

● Results indicate your blood glucose level at the precise time of testing.
● You can accurately measure a wide range of blood glucose levels (2-44 mmols/litre). Hypoglycaemia (level of blood sugar below 2.6 mmols/litre) can be measured and treated, as well as hyperglycaemia (above 6.6 mmols/litre).
● Measurement with this level of accuracy will enable you to solve particular problems, such as recurrent hypoglycaemic attacks which may occur at the same time each day.

Equipment

You will need to have:
● Reagent strips;
● Lancets or a finger pricking aid.
You may also wish to buy:
● A portable reflectance meter.

Reagent strips

Several different types of reagent strips are available, including:
BM Test Glycemie 1-44 (Boehringer Mannheim);
BM Test BG Strips (Boehringer Mannheim);
Glucostix (Ames);
Visidex II (Ames).

These are not available on prescription, and cost £7.00 — £8.50 for 50 sticks. With each stick the technique is slightly different and the manufacturer's instructions must be carefully followed for accuracy.

Lancets and finger-pricking aids

There are several devices available for pricking fingers to obtain a good drop of capillary blood without leaving a painful wound.

Examples of Finger Pricking Aids		Examples of Blood Lancets
Autoclix (Boehringer)	uses	Monolet Autoclix
Autolet (Owen Mumford)	uses	Monolet Unilet
Hypoguard Finger Pricker (Hypoguard)	uses	Any disposable ½" or ⅝" needles
Monojector (Monoject)	uses	Monoject
Glucolet (Ames)	uses	Unilet Monolet

Table 1. Finger pricking devices.
Finger pricking aids cost £4.00 — £10.00, and needles/lancets £3.00 — £8.00 per 100 (April 1986 prices).

Reflectance meters

There is a wide range of portable reflectance meters available. These make assessment of the colour on reagent strips easier and more accurate, but they are not available on prescription. Meters cost between £60.00 and £120.00.

Examples of Blood Glucose Meters

Glucocheck II (Medistron Ltd) (3 models, each for use with a different reagent strip). Can also be adapted to use sticks cut in half with a strip splitter (supplied by Medistron).

Glucometer (Ames) for use with Dextrostix.

Glucometer II (Ames) for use with Glucostix.

Talking Hypocount B (Hypoguard) for use with BM Test BG Strips (for blind people).

Table 2. Blood glucose meters.

Technique

Home blood glucose monitoring involves applying a good sized drop of capillary blood, usually from a finger prick, to a reagent strip. The blood is blotted or wiped off after a timed interval and a colour change develops during a further timed interval. The blood glucose result is read against a colour chart, or from a reflectance meter. Follow the directions on the diagram for the type of reagent strip you are using.

Causes of inaccurate readings include:
● Incorrect timing of procedure;
● Insufficient blood on the reagent strip;
● Out of date reagent strips left open to the air;
● Sweaty, dirty or "sugary" fingers;
● The reagent strip held wrong side up;
● Reflectance meter failure.

Check with your doctor or diabetic liaison nurse if you have any problems.

When and how often?

The answer to this depends on a variety of factors. Each person should work out a testing schedule with their doctor or diabetic liaison nurse. When learning how to achieve good diabetic control, or during alterations in treatment, testing may be required three or four times daily (before meals) to obtain a meaningful profile.

Once diabetic control is established testing may be carried out less frequently. If you have insulin dependent diabetes, extra "spot" tests are useful during periods of illness or unusual activity or rest when control may be temporarily lost. Because of fluctuations caused by exercise, food and timing of treatment, blood glucose is best measured at set times of the day so that results can be related to life events. Discuss this with your doctor or diabetic liaison nurse who may recommend measuring at a different time of day on each day of the week, repeated each week, or a full day's profile once or twice a week. If you have non-insulin dependent diabetes, regular testing over the day is not so important. A single fasting blood glucose can give a good idea of overall control throughout the day.

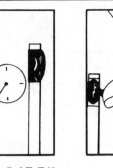

Good Blood Glucose Monitoring Technique

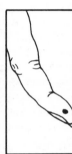

Always check with your doctor or diabetic liaison nurse if you have any problems.
He or she is ....
Telephone ....

There are three different techniques for monitoring blood glucose, depending on the type of reagent sticks you use. The first three steps are always the same:

1. Wash and dry hands. Do not use spirit on skin. Prick side or pulp of finger or thumb with suitable lancet.

2. Squeeze gently until large drop forms.

3. Turn hand until drop hangs from finger.

The next steps depend on your reagent sticks:

Technique for blood glucose testing using Visidex II.

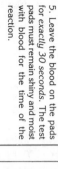

4. Apply blood freely to cover both reagent pads.

5. Leave the blood on the pads for exactly 30 seconds. The test pads must remain shiny and moist with blood for the time of the reaction.

6. Remove the blood either by blotting the strip once on absorbent tissue or by wiping the pads *gently* once or twice with a cotton wool ball. Wait an *additional 90 seconds* (2 minutes from applying the blood) before comparing pads to the colour charts.

Compare the green pad to the nearest matching green colour block. If the green block is darker than the 6 mmol/l colour block compare the lower pad to the nearest matching orange colour block. Record the result.

Techniques for blood glucose testing using BM Test Glycemie 1-44 R or BM Test BG strips.

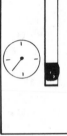 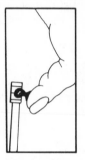

4. Touch blood on test pad. Do not spread or smear the blood.

5. Leave blood on test pad for *one minute.* This pad should be covered completely with the blood standing 'proud' on the strip.

6. Hold strip against a flat surface and wipe blood away *gently* three times with a clean pad of cotton wool.

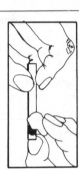

Leave test pad for one further minute and compare colour with label on tin or insert into meter.
When using *BM Test Glycemie 1-44* if the reading is at 2 minutes is above 13 mmol/l, leave for a further minute and read again.
When reading values below 7 mmol/l give priority to the lower blue test zone. For values above 7 mmol/l give priority to the block which matches the colour on the upper beige/green zone.
Record the result.

Technique for blood glucose testing using Dextrostix.

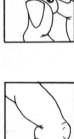

4. Turn hand until drop hangs from finger and apply blood freely to the entire reagent pad.

5. Time reaction for exactly *60 seconds.* The test pad must be completely covered and remain shiny and moist with blood for the time of the reaction. If only a thin film is spread over the area, throw the stick away and start again.

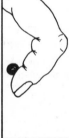

6. At one minute, immediately wash all the blood from the test strip with a sharp stream of water using a wash bottle directed just above the reagent area.

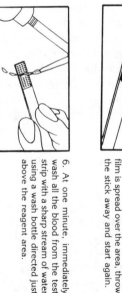

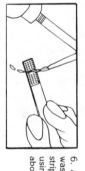 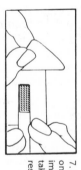

7. Blot the reagent pad of the strip on absorbent tissue. Insert immediately into the meter and take the reading. Record the result.

This handout is adapted from Sonksen, P. et al (1985) The Diabetes Reference Book, pp102-7, Harper and Row, London. The book is an excellent guide to coping with diabetes at home.
NB. The BM Test Glycemie 1-44 was until recently called BM Test Glycemie 20-800R.

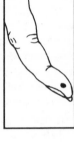
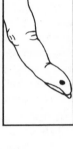

Living with a diabetic diet

Myra Ibbotson, BSc SRD
Freelance Dietitian

Until fairly recently, diabetic diets were quite drastic starvation-type regimens, usually based on restricting carbohydrate intake to less than 20-30 per cent of daily energy intake. This still continued even after insulin was introduced in 1921 because it was scarce and expensive.

Restricting carbohydrate intake had two consequences; first that people with diabetes avoided carbohydrates unnecessarily, and second, more seriously, that they depended too much on fat to provide their energy, which increased their chances of getting heart disease.

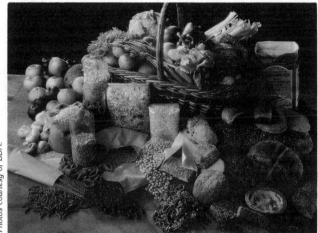

Choose high fibre foods like wholemeal bread, pasta and flour, and eat lots of fresh fruit and vegetables, either raw or lightly cooked to preserve their vitamins.

Photos courtesy of BDA.

Today's diabetic diet

The very restricted carbohydrate diet was recommended right up until 1982 when the British Diabetic Association (BDA) published an official policy statement which recommended several changes in the diabetic diet.

The BDA's recommendations allow greater carbohydrate intake while restricting fat intake and continuing to restrict sucrose and other simple sugars, though these are not necessarily completely avoided. They also put more emphasis on controlling total energy intake, so the recommendations are geared towards controlling all food intake instead of just restricting carbohydrate.

The 'new' diabetic diet is very similar to the diet that is now being recommended for the general population to reduce heart disease and generally improve health, which should mean that coping with a diabetic diet should get easier in future as consumer food manufacturers and suppliers become more aware of the need for suitable products.

Energy and carbohydrate intake

Your dietitian will advise you on how to organise your diet, based on your own personal needs. It is vital to control your energy (calorie) intake because evidence suggests that this is very important in long term control of diabetes.

Most hospitals recommend that about half of your energy comes from carbohydrate, and that two thirds of this is rich in fibre, which comes from wholemeal and wholegrain products, vegetables, pulses and fruits.

If you are receiving hypoglycaemic treatment — either insulin or tablets — it is important to time your carbohydrate intake carefully to avoid your blood sugar levels fluctuating too much. Your dietitian can advise you how to work an 'exchange system', which means that your meal plan can be more flexible.

Most people with diabetes who do not require other treatment are advised to lose weight, which means restricting energy intake. The new dietary recommendations make it easier to lose weight because you are less likely to get very hungry. You will be given a simple diet sheet containing meal plans and advice on cutting down on fat, salt and sugar. You should still see your dietitian regularly, as your dietary needs may change.

Fibre intake

The BDA recommends that people with diabetes eat 30g of mixed dietary fibre a day, which is what the rest of the population is also recommended to eat. This fibre both helps the gut to function and slows the absorption of sugar, which helps avoid sudden peaks in blood sugar. Some diabetic people have also reported having less hypoglycaemic (low blood sugar) incidences since going on a high fibre diet.

However, it is not just a question of eating fibre, because the type of fibre you eat, and the carbohydrate associated with it both have an additional effect. Fibres in beans or peas for instance (soluble fibres) have been found to reduce blood glucose levels after meals better than insoluble fibres such as wheat bran, starchy carbohydrates are released into the blood more slowly than sugary ones, so starchy, high fibre carbohydrates should make up most of your daily intake whatever medication you may be receiving.

Fat intake

The BDA recommends that fat intake is reduced to make up no more than 35 per cent of energy intake. Many people's intake is more than 40 per cent. Foods high in saturated fat should especially be avoided, to lessen the risk of arterial disease, but because this is a very long term aim, elderly people wit'. diabetes may not need to cut down their fat as much unless they need to lose weight.

Salt intake

People with diabetes are recommended to consume no more salt than those without the condition. This should not be too difficult to do as more people turn to a diet more reliant on cereals, fruit and vegetables and away from dairy produce and fatty meat products (especially the processed or manufactured ones like bacon, sausages and pies).

Alcohol

There is no reason to avoid alcohol if you have diabetes, but you should calculate its energy contribution. Also, hypoglycaemic incidences can look and feel like drunkenness when they are coming on, so you should be aware of the potential effects of alcohol so that you know what is affecting you, drink or your low blood sugar. Avoid sweet drinks like sweet sherry, port and liqueurs and if possible take alcohol with a meal. The low carbohydrate beers and lagers are both expensive and higher in alcohol and calories and so should be avoided. If you have no more than three drinks in one day (one drink is equal to half a pint of beer, one glass of wine or one measure of spirit) you can ignore the carbohydrate contribution. If you are overweight, however, you must still count the calories as part of your day's intake and not have more than one drink for every 1,000 calories a day you are allowed on your diet.

Putting recommendations into practice

● Change from low to high fibre foods.
This simply means choosing wholemeal rather than white products (eg bread, pasta, flour), having a high fibre breakfast cereal, and eating plenty of fruits and vegetables. Beans, peas or lentils should be included in soups, main dishes and salads regularly and these foods should provide about two thirds of the total carbohydrate content in any meal.

● Cut down on fat.
Choose low fat dairy produce, eat smaller portions of lean meat or other fatty 'protein' foods like cheese, use low fat cooking methods (eg stewing, braising, roasting, grilling) instead of frying, and avoid 'hidden' fat sources like pasties, cakes and biscuits.

● Eat regularly and space food intake across three or more meals.

● See the dietitian regularly.
Dietitians can help you adapt your eating habits and tailor an eating plan to your needs. They can also advise on how to distribute your food to tie in with your activity, lifestyle, medication and so on.

These changes are not easy to make on your own, but you should get plenty of help from the hospital or diabetes clinic. It is also well worth joining the BDA, who produce their own cookery books, advice sheets on a range of topics, a bi-monthly newspaper (Balance) and 'Countdown', a book detailing calorie and carbohydrate content of a wide range of proprietary products.

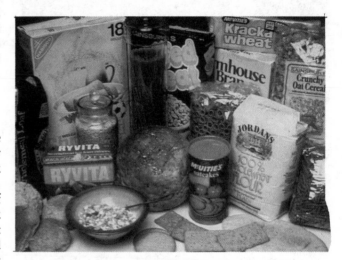

More and more proprietory brands of food are becoming suitable for a diabetic diet.

Diabetic products

There are many diabetic products on the market, but most are expensive and unnecessary. Most of the sweet products contain the same amount of calories as ordinary products. The most useful diabetic products are calorie free sweeteners like saccharine, aspartame and acesulfame K; low sugar or sugar free squashes and fizzy drinks and unsweetened products such as tinned fruit in fruit juice.

Special needs – illness

If you are unwell, have at least your normal insulin dose, balanced with an appropriate quantity of food. If you find this difficult, take carbohydrates in an easily managed form, in small quantities across the day if necessary (see Table 1).

Table 1. Exchange list for illness (each exchange = 10g carbohydrate).

2 teaspoons sugar/glucose. 50mls Lucozade. 100mls cola (coke) drink. 30mls neat ordinary fruit squash. 200mls milk (= 1 average glass). 1 small brickette ice cream. 200mls thick tinned soup.

Exercise

Regular exercise is as good for you as for anyone else, but it will have to be accounted for in your diet plan. If you take vigorous and unscheduled exercise, you may need to 'top up' with about 20g of carbohydrate beforehand. If appetite or time are limited, a mini Mars or Milky Way bar; three to six dextrose tablets, a cereal snack bar or chocolate biscuit are acceptable. This can also be a way of giving children sweet treats without disturbing their diabetic control. If you take prolonged exercise, you may need more 'top-ups', and you may also need extra carbohydrates at your next meal or snack to prevent hypoglycaemia. A list of 10g 'top-ups' is in Table 2.

Available from the BDA

Food values lists
Countdown (guide to the nutritional value of manufactured products)
Simple Diabetic Recipes
Simple Home Baking
Better Cookery for Diabetics
Cooking the Diabetic Way (for those trying to lose weight)
Packed Lunches and Snacks
The Diabetic's Microwave Cookbook

For further information about these and other BDA publications, write to: The British Diabetic Association, 10 Queen Anne Street, London W1N 0BD.

Suggested further reading

The Diabetic's Diet Book, by J.I. Mann and the Oxford Dietetic Group. Published by Martin Dunitz.
Diabetic Medicine (1984) by J.I. Mann in *Diabetic Medicine*, **1**, 191-8.

These are both useful if you are interested in finding out more about the diabetic diet.

Table 2. Exchange list (each item = 10g carbohydrate or 1 exchange).

The foods marked * are high in fibre and low in fat, and should comprise ⅔ of the daily carbohydrate intake. Use a standard kitchen measuring spoon.

Bread	1 slice from small wholemeal loaf* 1 slice from small white loaf ½ average sized chapati*
Biscuits	1 large digestive* 2 semisweet biscuits, eg Rich Tea, Marie 2 wholegrain crispbreads*
Rice/Pasta	3 heaped tablespoons brown rice or wholewheat pasta (cooked)* 2 tablespoons wholemeal flour*
Breakfast Cereals	1 Weetabix* ⅔ Shredded Wheat* 4-5 tablespoons All-Bran, Branflakes* 4-5 tablespoons Cornflakes 4 tablespoons cooked porridge (or 15g using raw oats)*
Fruit	1 average orange, apple, pear or peach* 2 tangerines* 1 small banana* 15g dried fruit, eg sultanas* 100ml glass unsweetened fruit juice
Vegetables	1 egg sized boiled or jacket potato* 50-75g cooked pulses, eg lentils, haricot beans, butter beans* 4-5 tablespoons sweetcorn* 4 tablespoons baked beans* Most other vegetables can be eaten freely.
Miscellaneous	2 large sausages, 2 fish fingers, 3 teaspoons malted milk beverage

One of the first skills that the insulin-dependent patient has to learn in order to be self-sufficient is injection technique, and the nurse is required to make sure that the patient understands and can demonstrate correct preparation and injection of the insulin.

Injection techniques:
Teaching diabetic patients

Sheila Reading, BSc, SRN
Diabetes Research Sister, Dept. of Primary Medical Care, Southampton University

As long ago as 1924, Edward Joslin referring to the person with diabetes wrote ". . . education of the patient to care for himself constitutes 90 per cent of the treatment".

Injection technique is one of the first skills that the insulin-dependent patient needs to learn in order to be self sufficient. Traditionally it is the nurse, either in hospital or the community, who is called on to take responsibility for teaching this practical aspect of care, and in her role as educator an understanding of the teaching-learning process is necessary (Coutts and Hardy, 1985).

Patients close to the time of diagnosis of their disorder are often distressed and even overwhelmed by their new condition; but simply giving the patient time to voice concerns about diabetes or the injection before the injection lesson may do much to create the trusting situation in which a patient can best learn. Individual needs, abilities, and motivation to learn must be assessed to help the patient understand and demonstrate correct preparation of the insulin injection and proper injection technique. The baseline for each patient's understanding of their new needs will be different, and this will also need careful assessment by the nurse to enable her to teach at an appropriate level and from the right starting point for each individual.

Arrangements should be made for the nurse to be present at several injections until the patient is confident at all stages: choosing the insulin dose, drawing it up, and injecting it, and caring for the equipment. A visit timed for after the injection to check that all went well is a good way of "handing over" to the patient.

Points to consider when teaching the injection technique

- Keep the procedure simple.
- Arrange sessions to involve members of the patient's family.
- Give support and clear explanation from the outset to prevent bad habits developing, eg poor mixing of insulins, poor choice of sites, skin blebbing.
- Make sure all the professionals involved are agreed on teaching the same technique. Patients lose confidence if they receive conflicting advice.
- Provide teaching aids as a back-up facility. Literature can be read at the patient's leisure, eg "Knowing about Diabetes: Insulin-dependent Diabetics" (Wise, 1983).
- Explain the theoretical concepts underlying each step in the procedure.
- Allow time for questions to be asked.
- Remember to give praise and encouragement.
- Evaluate the success of the teaching.

References
Coutts, L. C., and Hardy, L. K., (1985) Teaching for Health: The Nurse as Health Educator. Churchill Livingstone.
Joslin, E. P., (1924). The Treatment of Diabetes Mellitus (3rd edition). Henry Kempton, London.
Wise, P. H., (1983). Knowing about Diabetes: For Insulin-dependent Diabetics. W. Foulsham and Co. Ltd., London.

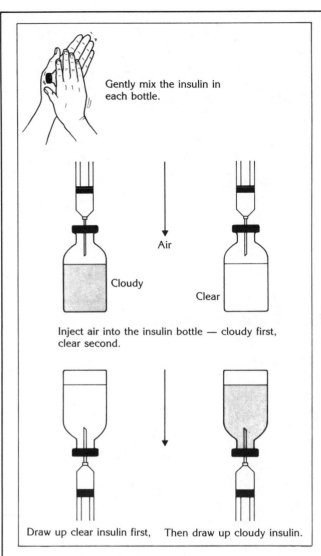

Figure 1. Drawing up a mixed dose injection.

Drawing up insulin
1. Don't keep the current insulin bottle in the fridge or injections will feel cold.
2. Gently mix the contents of the insulin bottle by rolling it between the palms of your hands. Do not shake vigorously because this will cause the insulin to froth.
3. Draw back the plunger of the syringe to introduce air, and inject it into the insulin bottle. Injection of as many units of air into the insulin bottle as the number to be withdrawn prevents a vacuum from forming.
   This makes it easier to draw insulin into the syringe without bubbles.
4. With the needle still inserted, invert the bottle and check that the needle is below the surface of the insulin.
   Holding the syringe at eye level, slowly draw up the insulin. If any bubbles develop flick the side of syringe and move the plunger in and out until the correct dose of insulin, minus bubbles, is in the syringe. Withdraw the needle, and proceed to inject the insulin.

Drawing up a mixed dose injection (Figure 1)
If clear (short acting, eg Actrapid) and cloudy (intermediate or long acting, eg Monotard) insulins are to be mixed, inject air into the *cloudy* insulin bottle first. Withdraw the needle and then inject air into the *clear* insulin bottle and proceed to draw up the required dose of clear insulin. Finally reinsert the needle into the bottle of cloudy insulin and withdraw the correct dose.

Always draw up insulin from the clear bottle first to avoid contamination from the cloudy insulin.

If too much cloudy insulin is drawn up by mistake, it is safest to expel all the mixture in the syringe into a sink and start again.

Sites for insulin injection
Insulin can be injected wherever there is enough subcutaneous tissue. The most suitable sites are therefore the thighs, abdomen, arms, and buttocks (See Figure 2).

It is important to vary the point of injection each time, because continued use of one site can lead to it becoming hard, lumpy, and in time devoid of sensation. Should this happen, the site must not be used for injecting. The absorption of insulin from such an area can become erratic.

Injection technique
Insulin should be injected 20-30 minutes before a meal in order to give it time to act before the patient eats.
1. The skin need not be specially cleaned if you bathe regularly. Repeated application of spirit hardens the skin and may cause stinging when the needle carries it through the skin.
2. Check the dose of insulin drawn up in the syringe, and choose a site for injecting. (See Figure 2).
3. Pinch a generous fold of skin between the thumb and finger of one hand, and holding the syringe like a dart in the other, quickly insert the needle at about 75-90 degrees to the skin. The needle should be pushed in almost to the hilt and the insulin smoothly injected.
4. Withdraw the needle. If there is any leakage from the injection site press a clean tissue or pad of cotton wool to it for a few seconds.

Gently mix the insulin in each bottle.

Air

Cloudy

Clear

Inject air into the insulin bottle — cloudy first, clear second.

Draw up clear insulin first,   Then draw up cloudy insulin.

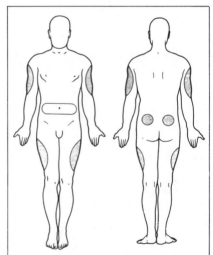

Figure 2. Sites for injection.

Bibliography

Drawing and Injecting Insulin. (1982) Becton-Dickinson UK Ltd., Consumer Products Division, Between Towns Road, Cowley, Oxford OX4 3LY.
   Step-by-step presentation of procedure intended for use with diabetic patients. Includes 27 colour slides and notes.
Kinson, J., and Nattrass, M., (1984) Caring for the Diabetic Patient. Churchill Livingstone.
   This book provides an understanding of diabetes mellitus and much practical advice.
Wilson-Barnett, J., (1983) Editor. Recent Advances in Nursing: Patient Teaching. Churchill Livingstone.
   Includes a chapter entitled "Teaching the diabetic patient" (by Marks, C.) This text deals with aspects of education for a variety of client groups.

The above guidelines may be useful for patients. However, slight variations in policy do exist.

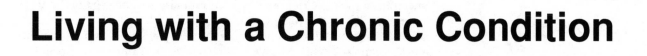

Living with a Chronic Condition

The new stroke victim may face a dramatic change of life-style which could have far-reaching effects on the lives of carers. This Patient Education Plus offers some ideas on the information, education and support they may require.

Mobility problems of the new stroke victim: Supporting the carer

Elizabeth M. Horne, MA
Editorial Director, The Professional Nurse

Patients and relatives will vary considerably in their levels of awareness of the nature of a stroke and its effect on mobility, in their understanding of its effects on different faculties and the contribution they can make in helping the stroke victim regain mobility. The nurse's level of language and detail when explaining the nature and effects of the stroke will therefore need to be carefully chosen for each person. It is essential for the carer to have some understanding of the complexity of mobility problems, including all the factors outlined in Table 1.

Motivation

A major source of concern for a new stroke victim's carers is the uncertainty over the degree to which mobility will be regained and the length of time that rehabilitation will take. Both will vary considerably between patients, depending on age, severity of stroke and personality, but the carers should be given plenty of opportunity to express their anxieties, and as much information as possible about the likely pattern of rehabilitation for that person.

Rehabilitation may be very slow, and the degree of disability will probably vary from day to day, causing frustration and uncertainty and undermining the patient's self-confidence.

Perceptual problems, and poor memory or concentration span may make the patient appear to lack motivation about rehabilitation. An understanding of these by the carer may ease the frustrations of rehabilitation.

The stroke victim may be reluctant to use aids, feeling they represent an admission of disability. By encouraging discussion of this issue with the stroke victim and the carers, the nurse can help the stroke victim to come to terms with the new situation, and the carer to understand the patient's feelings more fully.

Basic points in assisting mobility

The carer may need a considerable amount of detailed practical help and advice from the doctor, physiotherapist, and occupational therapist on the correct positioning, methods of lifting and moving the patient, on exercises to promote rehabilitation and on the availability and use of appropriate aids, furniture and appliances in the home.

This advice and information should be followed up by the nurse, to ensure that the carer knows how to use the aids, and is confident about using them. The future carer should be fully involved with moving the stroke victim while still in hospital: watching the nurses, and then actually manoeuvering the patient under nursing supervision. Encouragement from the nurses can be invaluable in building up the future carer's self-confidence.

While encouraging the patient to be independent in hospital, the nurse will also need to recognise the patient's areas of difficulty and try to prevent him or her becoming tired and discouraged. Future carers should also be encouraged to follow this pattern. If the patient becomes too dependent on others, there may be less incentive to acquire the skills he or she will need to fully develop their mobility.

Importance of individual assessment

The new stroke victim and carers should be involved in assessing present skills and setting realistic goals in rehabilitation. The assessment of the home environment is also essential and must involve all relevant members of the household in conjunction with all members of the community-based caring team, including nurses, the GP, community physiotherapist and community occupational therapist, the speech therapist and also social services. Mobility aids, and adaptations required to a bathroom or kitchen may be available from social services, but could take some considerable time to arrange. Information about commercially available aids and furniture may be helpful.

Continuing support

Carers should be encouraged to remember their own health and strength over the coming months. They may welcome information on locally or nationally organized support groups, and may benefit from meeting people in similar situations. The social services should be able to provide information about local schemes to enable the carer to take a holiday.

Where further day hospital or outpatient care is envisaged, the patient and carers could be introduced to the relevant staff before discharge from hospital.

Regular contact with the community care team should involve the continuing assessment and setting of new goals in the rehabilitation programme.

The handout overleaf can be photocopied for distribution to patients and carers, and may form a useful starting point for the programme of rehabilitation.

Because of the high incidence of speech impairment suffered by stroke victims, it is important that carers communicate on their behalf with the authorities to ensure they receive the benefits to which they are entitled.

Useful contacts:

District nurse:
Community occupational therapist:
Community physiotherapist:
Speech therapist:
Day hospital or outpatients:
Social worker:
Local stroke club:
Local transport scheme:

**The Chest, Heart & Stroke Association (CHSA)
Tavistock House North,
Tavistock Square, London WC1H 9JE
Tel: 01-387 3012**

Scotland: 65 North Castle Street
Edinburgh EH2 3LT
Tel: 031-225 6963

Northern Ireland: 28 Bedford Street
Belfast BT2 7FJ
Tel: 0232-220184

The CHSA works for the prevention of chest, heart and stroke illnesses and to help those who suffer from them. They publish a number of useful publications.

**The Disabled Living Foundation (DLF)
380 — 384 Harrow Road
London W9 2HU
Tel: 01-289 6111**

The DLF is concerned with those aspects of ordinary life which present particular problems to disabled people of any age. They have set up an aids and equipment centre displaying aids for disabled people and run a valuable information service. They publish a number of useful publications.

**Action for Dysphasic Adults
Northcote House, 37a Royal Street
London SE1 7LL
Tel: 01-261 9572**

ADA publishes leaflets for adults with speech impairment and their carers and campaigns to get speech therapy for stroke victims.

**Disability Alliance Education & Research Association
21 Star Street, London W2 1QB, or
25 Denmark Street, London WC2**

The Alliance provides a service to disabled people and their carers on disability benefits available. They publish the Disability Rights Handbook (price £2.40).

Table 1: Factors affecting mobility in the stroke patient

Impairment	Effect on mobility
Hemiparesis or hemiplegia	Innervation of muscles of legs, trunk and arms may be lost, causing paralysis.
Visual disturbances Perceptual difficulties Balance problems (if cerebellum has been affected)	Balance will be affected if vision, or the processing by the brain of visual information, or the balancing functions of the cerebellum are affected.
Communication	Impairment of speech, or of cognitive or reasoning functions may indirectly affect mobility if the stroke victim is unable to communicate his or her plans, intentions or wishes related to movement. Embarrassment over impaired ability to communicate may inhibit the person's progress toward mobility.
Psychological and social	Fear, anxiety and depression associated with the patient's changed body image will result in some loss of self-confidence which could affect the person's confidence in mobility. The initial uncertainty about the nature of the new patterns of mobility will also knock this self confidence.
Environmental	A once-familiar home may have become an obstacle-course for the new stroke victim, with steps and stairways and narrow doorways which may present insuperable barriers to reasonable mobility.

The care of the new stroke victim

Mobility

Complete this form with the help of your nurse:

Patient assessment: The stroke caused particular problems because it affected:

Movement: Vision:

Balance: Perception:

Objectives

We aim to be able to do the following tasks by...1986:

....

Carer   **Patient**

Some points for the carer to bear in mind

- Make sure you are confident about moving and positioning the patient correctly. Ask the nurse or physiotherapist to show you the correct way to work with the patient while he or she is still in hospital, and to let you try with their supervision. Always ask if you are not sure, or if you would like more help. There is an excellent booklet called 'Home care for the stroke patient in the early days' available from the Chest, Heart & Stroke Association, price 60p, which gives clear details on positioning and moving the patient, and on the exercises they may need to do.
- Make sure that the patient wears appropriate clothing and footwear. Avoid slippers or loose shoes, and very loose clothing. Your own footwear is important, too, if you are involved in lifting or helping the patient to move.
- Work out, with your district nurse and community occupational therapist, what would be the most valuable aids and appliances in the home. Are there any adaptations (such as grip-rails near the bath, or replacement of soft carpeting with firmer floor coverings) which you could see to yourself, or ask a friend or relative to fix? Ask your community occupational therapist about the best kind of chairs and beds and their availability.
- Make sure you know how to use all the aids and appliances fully and correctly. Ask your district nurse or community occupational therapist if you are not sure.
- Check regularly that all the aids are safe: look for worn ferrules on walking sticks and check the heels of shoes for uneven wear.
- Try not to let the patient become discouraged when he or she is tired, or frustrated. Rehabilitation may be slow, and his or her apparent degree of disability may vary from day to day. It may also take him or her some time to come to terms with the new situation.
- Don't lose sight of your *own* health. Caring for a stroke victim may be hard work both physically and emotionally, and your own good health is an essential requirement.
- Make contact with your local stroke association and national organizations. Your district nurse should be able to help you here.
- Find out about local transport schemes, exemption from vehicle excise duty, and mobility allowance, and the orange badge scheme. Information should be available from Social Services.

There is no reason why people with chronic respiratory disease should have to endure a poor quality of life once they have been discharged from hospital. This chapter describes a patient education programme implemented on the ward prior to the patient's discharge.

Living with lung problems

Pauline Bagnall, RGN
Respiratory Health Worker, Department of Medicine, Charing Cross Hospital, London

Janice Sigsworth, RGN
Sister, University College Hospital, London

Chronic respiratory disease is the single most common condition causing disability between the ages of 35 and 74 years (Bennett and Halil, 1970). Chronic bronchitis, emphysema and asthma are responsible for over 0.5 million periods of sickness absence from work per annum, a 10 per cent occupancy of hospital medical beds (Royal College of Physicians, 1981). People with chronic respiratory disease can now be kept alive longer because of effective treatment for infections and episodes of respiratory failure. However, their quality of life may be poor – breathlessness has both a physical and psychological impact upon the individual and the family.

A working party of the Royal College of Physicians recognised the need to pay attention to long-term care as well as 'crisis intervention' and its report (1981) recommended the creation of Respiratory Health Workers (RHWs) to support and educate the patient following discharge, in an attempt to increase knowledge, reduce hospitalisation and improve the quality of the patient's life. A controlled trial in Charing Cross Hospital (Cockcroft, Bagnall, Heslop et al, 1986) attempted to follow the report's recommendations and to measure the effectiveness of nurse intervention. Results showed that patients visited by the RHW increased their knowledge of their condition and medications in comparison with the control group.

Maintaining a safe environment
Communication
Breathing
Eating and drinking
Eliminating
Personal cleansing and dressing
Controlling body temperature
Mobilising
Working and playing
Expressing sexuality
Sleeping
Dying

Table 1. Activities of living.

Health education within a nursing framework

Bagnall and Heslop (1987) recommended that teaching programmes should be introduced in hospital before discharge, to be continued by community nurses. Superimposing health education upon conventional medical and nursing care, a patient education programme has now been started on a general medical ward specialising in respiratory medicine. The system of implementing a programme of health education is supported by the use of a nursing model (Roper, Logan and Tierney,

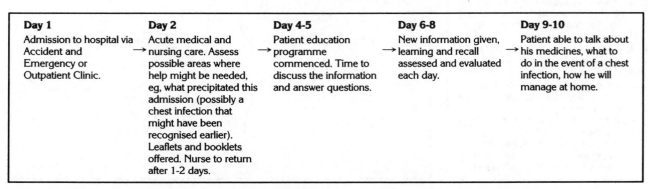

Day 1	Day 2	Day 4-5	Day 6-8	Day 9-10
Admission to hospital via Accident and Emergency or Outpatient Clinic.	Acute medical and nursing care. Assess possible areas where help might be needed, eg, what precipitated this admission (possibly a chest infection that might have been recognised earlier). Leaflets and booklets offered. Nurse to return after 1-2 days.	Patient education programme commenced. Time to discuss the information and answer questions.	New information given, learning and recall assessed and evaluated each day.	Patient able to talk about his medicines, what to do in the event of a chest infection, how he will manage at home.

Figure 1. Flow chart to demonstrate when the teaching/learning takes place in relation to a patient's stay in hospital.

1. Problem: Mr K does not know about his lung disease and how to cope with it at home.
Goal: Mr K will tell me how his lung disease affects him and his life before discharge.
Plan: 20.5.87 Leaflets and booklets given.
21.5.87 Discussion about anatomy and physiology of lungs and how lung disease affects Mr K's life.
25.5.87 Mr K is able to tell me how lung disease affects his body and his life.

Table 2. Part of an education plan.

1983). This model examines the individual's performance within the activities of living (Table 1) and provides a framework which demonstrates clearly the ways nurses can interact purposefully with patients. The nursing process is also implemented on the ward: "a diagnostic and management tool which promotes problem solving, critical thinking, care planning, analysis and data collecting" (Darcy, 1980).

On admission, patients are assessed in terms of their daily living activities (DLA), problems are identified and goals set. The patient's care is planned according to the set goals; evaluation of the patient's progress is a continuous process. Patient care is managed through a modified system of primary nursing (Sparrow, 1986) in which 22 patients are grouped into three management units. Each unit is managed by two to three Registered General Nurses (RGNs) – the primary nurses. Each primary nurse is responsible for between six and eight patients from admission to discharge, incorporating the assessment, planning, giving and evaluating of nursing care to meet the individual needs of the patients.

The education programme

As soon as it is practicable, for example, when the acute stage of the illness is over (Figure 1) patients are asked by the primary nurse if they would like some information about their lung disease and help to understand and cope with it. Initially they are given relevant leaflets and booklets to read. A contract is made with the patient for the nurse to return at a specified time a day or two later to discuss the information and answer any queries; they usually find it helpful to write questions down before the nurse returns.

From this initial brief discussion the nurse can usually elicit where the main areas of concern lie. Education needs include understanding lung disease and how it affects the patient's life; understanding the uses and side-effects of medicines, including home nebulisers and oxygen therapy; how to reach a stated goal weight, stop smoking and resume an active life. Further appointments to see the patient are made depending on these needs and the amount of teaching and learning that is required. Individual education plans using the problem-solving process (as identified above) are used and inserted into the nursing Kardex. Table 2 illustrates part of one patient's teaching programme.

1. Patient is to define the basic components of the respiratory and cardiac systems.
2. Patient is to say how his lung disease affects his lungs.
3. Patient is to say how he will recognise and describe the symptoms of breathlessness and relate these to his own breathless episodes.
4. Patient is to say what the signs and symptoms of a chest infection or health deterioration may be and what action he will take.
5. Demonstrate self-use (or carer) of oxygen equipment.
6. Demonstrate how to use a home nebuliser or inhaler(s).
7. Participate in self-administration of medicines and say the names, actions and side-effects of each one.

Table 3. Checklist of competencies.

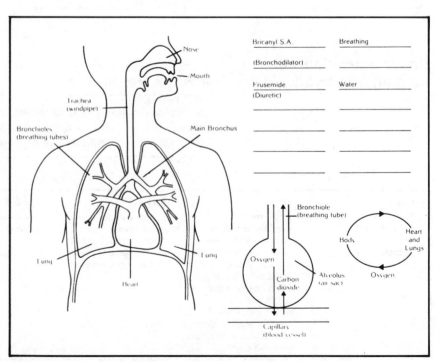

Figure 2. The teaching aid given to patients.

The work is structured on individual patient care and the education plans are tailored to individual needs so that each person is taught as much or as little as they want to know. A checklist of areas that nursing staff like people to be competent in before discharge is kept on the ward (Table 3). However during the RHW project Bagnall and Heslop (1987) found that education is not always of primary importance to the person concerned. Nurses must be sensitive to the needs and priorities that *patients* think are important and must not underestimate that patients probably do not feel well.

A continuous process

Not all teaching takes place at 'specific' times, it is a continuous process. For example, Mr B does not know how to use his inhaler correctly. The primary nurse would identify this as a problem and spend some time explaining why it is important to use the inhaler properly. She would also demonstrate the correct technique with a placebo inhaler, and this interaction would be documented on the teaching plan. The primary nurse would ask the other nurses looking after Mr B to supervise, monitor and record his progress on the care plan at each drug round. The primary nurse is then able to evaluate Mr B's progress when she returns to continue the teaching plan.

Relatives and people important to the patient are involved wherever possible. The teaching aid designed for the RHW study (Bagnall and Heslop, 1987) is used and given to patients to keep (Figure 2). It is usually easier to describe the anatomy and physiology with both anatomical and colloquial names (for example, the alveoli are often referred to as air sacs). A factsheet is also given to the patient (see handout). Health education authority leaflets about asthma, lung disease, diet, smoking, hypertension and exercise are used wherever possible to supplement teaching. There are two education boards in each corridor of the ward displaying relevant information. The patients are encouraged to read and ask questions about this information to improve their knowledge of their condition.

Patient goals

Before discharge it is hoped that each patient has reached his stated goals. For some people this may be demonstrating knowledge in each of the areas on the checklist. For others it may be saying when they should be taking their medicines.

This patient education programme is still in an embryonic stage. An index is kept of all the patients who receive the education programme, along with copies of their education plans so that the programme can be updated continually and the style revised. Nurses need knowledge to be able to give knowledge. A group of primary nurses are following the distance learning pack on patient education (organised and run by the Polytechnic of the South Bank) in order to develop and improve their skills as educators.

These authors would like to evaluate the programme – goal analysis will be used and possible audit of the care plans. At present, one of the best evaluations to hand is that patients do seem to enjoy and appreciate their new knowledge. The long-term goal would be to continue the education process in the patient's home. The primary nurse would then be responsible for the patient's education from admission through to, and following, discharge until the patients can say that they have sufficient knowledge to live a good quality of life, and to maintain health.

The aim of health education and patient teaching is to equip people intellectually and emotionally for making sound decisions on matters affecting their health and welfare (Clark and Webb, 1985). We believe our patient education programme goes some way towards giving patients the choice and right to know how to cope with their lung disease at home. The handout overleaf can be freely photocopied for distribution to patients and clients.

References

Bagnall, P. and Heslop, A. (1987) Chronic respiratory disease: Educating patients at home. *The Professional Nurse,* 2, 9, 293-6.

Bennett, A.E. and Halil, T. (1970) Chronic disease and disability in the community: A prevalence study. *BMJ,* 3, 762-4.

Clarke, J.M. and Webb, P. (1985) Health education – a basis for professional nursing practice. *Nursing Education Today,* 5, 210-214.

Cockcroft, A. et al (1986) Controlled trial of a respiratory health worker visiting patients with chronic respiratory disability. *BMJ,* 294, 225-8.

Darcy, P.T. (1980) The nursing process – a base for all nursing developments. *Nursing Times,* 76, 497-501.

Polytechnic of the South Bank. Teaching patients and clients (Distance Learning Package).

Roper, N., Logan, W. and Tierney, A. (1983) Using a Model for Nursing. Churchill-Livingstone, Edinburgh.

Royal College of Physicians (1981) Disabling chest disease: Prevention and care. *J. Royal Coll. of Physicians,* 15, 2, 69-87.

Sparrow, S. (1986) Primary nursing. *Nursing Practice,* 1, 142-8.

So You've Got Lung Problems?

We have one right and one left lung. In between these is the heart. We breathe in air which contains oxygen. Oxygen is vital for life. The air travels through the nose and mouth, down the trachea (windpipe) and into each lung. It then travels along the bronchial tree (breathing tubes) to the alveoli (air sacs). The oxygen passes from the air sacs to the bloodstream. This oxygenated blood is pumped by the heart to the body. Carbon dioxide is a waste product from the body and is exchanged with the oxygen in the blood so that it can be breathed out.

What can go wrong?

Chronic bronchitis The air passages of the lungs become swollen and narrow. An excess of phlegm (sputum) is produced. This leads to breathlessness and the coughing up of sputum, especially in the morning.

Emphysema The walls between the air sacs break down leading to fewer, larger air sacs. This leads to breathlessness because the area through which oxygen passes from the air sac to the bloodstream has been reduced.

Asthma The breathing tubes become narrow and inflamed which leads to breathlessness and wheezing.

Bronchiectasis An excess amount of sputum is produced, leading to breathlessness.

What will the doctor do?

The doctor will examine you and take a history. He or she may order some tests including a chest X-ray, lung function tests (which involve blowing into a machine several times) and blood tests. He or she will then decide on the most appropriate treatment for you.

Medicines

Bronchodilators eg, Salbutamol, (Ventolin), terbutaline (Bricanyl). They dilate (open up) the breathing tubes to allow air to enter and leave the lungs. They may be prescribed either as tablets, inhalers or nebuliser solutions.

Steroids eg, Prednisolone, Becotide, Becloforte. They help to reduce the swelling of the walls of the breathing tubes and therefore also help to allow air in and out of the lungs. Prednisolone is available as tablets, Becotide and Becloforte as inhalers.

Diuretics eg, Frusemide, Amiloride. They help to get rid of excess water within the body. This helps the heart to work more effectively and therefore to pump oxygenated blood around the body. They are available as tablets.

Antibiotics eg, Septrin, Ampicillin, Amoxycillin. They are prescribed when a chest infection is present. It is important to complete the course of antibiotics so that the chest infection is cleared up completely. They are prescribed as tablets.

Oxygen Some people may need oxygen at home to help them breathe more easily. It may be supplied in cylinders or as an oxygen concentrator (a machine that concentrates oxygen from the surrounding air).

When should you take medical advice?

When your lungs are damaged you become more susceptible to having chest infections. It is important that these infections are treated promptly to minimise the risk of reducing your lung function further. One of the first signs of a chest infection is that your sputum changes colour. Sputum is normally white or clear. If it becomes green or yellow a chest infection is present; you may also be feeling more breathless than usual. When this occurs it is important to start taking a course of antibiotics immediately. Either contact your GP, who will prescribe a course, or, if you have a reserve supply of antibiotics at home, start the course yourself. If your sputum remains discoloured when you have finished the course, and you feel no better, tell your doctor – a further course or another type of antibiotic may be

How do you help yourself to stay well?

1. Take adequate exercise to improve your breathing circulation and general wellbeing. Feeling breathless is frightening but, it is not dangerous, and small amounts of regular exercise will help to make you feel much better.

2. Eat a balanced diet. If you are overweight then try to lose some weight to lessen the load on your heart and lungs.

3. Do not smoke – smoke acts as an irritant to your lungs. Cigarette smoking is known to damage the lungs.

4. Try to get 7 or 8 hours sleep in 24 hours – not necessarily at night.

5. Take your medicines as prescribed and in the correct manner so full benefit will be gained from them.

6. Check the colour of your sputum every day. If it changes colour start a course of antibiotics (a course may be for 5, 7 or 10 days, depending on the type of antibiotic prescribed). Remember to complete the whole course.

I hope this fact sheet has been useful and answered some of your questions. If you have any further ones it may be a good idea to jot them down on a piece of paper so you will remember them when I next see you.

Contact ....

Telephone No. ....

Intermittent self-catheterisation can enable certain groups of incontinent people to lead active lives.

Self-catheterisation – a solution for some incontinent people

Philip McSweeney, MA, Cert Ed, Dip N, SRN
Senior Tutor/Senior Lecturer, North East Essex School of Nursing, Colchester

Intermittent self-catheterisation (ISC) is becoming more widely used. Not only does it enable patients to lead a more active or 'normal' life, but it can also resolve many of the demoralising problems associated with incontinence, such as permanently wearing pads or aids.

ISC can be used in situations where the client's bladder can contain a reasonable volume of urine before leakage occurs or the bladder voids spontaneously. As a reasonable guide, if the patient can remain continent following emptying of the bladder by catheter for over two hours, he or she can establish a pattern of appropriate times to self-catheterise. A frequency of four to six times per day is usual.

Which patients?

The technique is better suited to patients with an underactive detrusor function and a 'high compliance' bladder (capacious, with little change in pressure) (ICS, 1981) and/or an overactive urethral closure mechanism. Both these conditions imply a neuropathic deficit and both can be detected or implied by urodynamic studies (Torrens, 1987).

Patient groups for whom the technique has been documented include those whose conditions have obvious neuropathic cause, such as spinal nerve damage (Youngjohns, 1984; Winder, 1986) eg, paraplegia following trauma; spina bifida cystica or occulta (Youngjohns, 1984), especially children (Deegan, 1985); and multiple sclerosis (Youngjohns, 1984; Winder, 1986; Blannin, 1986). In a study by Murray et al (1984), the most common indication for ISC was chronic urine retention.

ISC helps prevent the long-term complications associated with chronic retention and protects the renal system. Deegan further documents how the technique has been used for patients with previous urinary diversion who have been 'undiverted'; those who have had micturition delayed by drug therapy and those who have had their bladder capacity surgically increased (colocystoplasty).

Bibliography
Mandelstam, D. (ed) (1986) Incontinence and its Management. Croom Helm, London.
A useful handbook of reference material.
Norton, C. (1986) Nursing for Continence. Beaconsfield Pub. Ltd, Beaconsfield.
A significant, practical guide for nurses.
Simcare ISC information booklets for the family, patient and nurse. Eschmann Bros and Walsh Ltd, Lancing, West Sussex.
Wilson-Barnett, J. (ed) (1983) Patient Teaching. Churchill Livingstone, Edinburgh.
Reviews important issues in patient teaching.

Assessment

References
Ausubel, D. (1968) Education Psychology – A cognitive view. Holt, Rinehart and Winston, New York.
Blannin, J. (1986) My Three D's. Coloplast Supplement on Continence Promotion. *Nursing*, 10.
Deegan, S. (1985) Intermittent catheterisation for children. *Nursing Times*, **81**, 14, 72–74.

continued overleaf

Where possible, the cause of incontinence needs to be known, as it may preclude initiatives such as habit training or pelvic floor exercises. In such cases, it may help to determine suitability if the patient keeps a continence chart to determine the incontinence pattern. Other factors need to be considered during assessment – a list is given in Table 1 overleaf.

These factors need to be considered with the patient. As a physical skill, the technique is not difficult – what seems paramount to success is the patient's motivation. Any reluctance on the part of the patient – or the partner or parent – is usually more to do with the apparently undignified nature of the procedure than a physical impediment. It is important, therefore, to encourage the patient and partner to talk about their feelings and demonstrate an emphathic response.

The 'clean' technique

A technique that is clean, as opposed to aseptic, has been described by a number of authors (Lapides et al, 1972; Youngjohns, 1984), and can be taught to patients in hospital or at home. The risk of introducing infection is kept low by the clean procedure, minimal time of catheter in bladder and by encouraging over two litres of fluid intake per day.

In a study by Murray et al (1984) 30 out of 57 ISC patients followed for up to five years provided a CSU for microscopy. None had pathological bacteriuria, though 43 per cent had coliforms present. No prophylactic antibiotics were given and symptomatic urinary infection was treated on the basis of antibiotic sensitivities.

Which catheters?

1. Does the cause render 'retraining' initiatives inappropriate?
2. Is the patient aware of the range of choice over continence management?
3. Is the number of times the patient would have to self-catheterise to maintain continence realistic?
4. Does the patient understand the technique and its relative advantages/disadvantages?
5. Does the patient seem motivated to learn?
6. What is the patient's physical capacity to perform the technique? Consider manual dexterity, degree of handicap eg, vision, extent of paralysis, ability to get in a position to achieve access to the urethra, especially female patients.
7. What support/assistance/environment will the patient have? A partner may perform the technique if acceptable to both.

Table 1. Factors to consider in patient assessment for ISC.

In selecting catheters it is important to consider a number of points.
- The diameter need only be about 12FG for an adult, 8FG for a child.
- The catheter material, especially the tip, needs to be fairly rigid, but with smooth drainage eyes to prevent urethral trauma.
- Male and female catheter lengths can be used; alternatively, suction catheters may suffice and may also be cheaper.
- Choose catheters available on FP10.

Good teaching with two-way interaction should enable patients to cope better and it is essential to establish a rapport with the patient at the outset. Poor patient teaching is often marked by a lack of any structured approach, but teaching can follow the steps of the nursing process.

An assessment of what needs to be taught should begin with Ausubel's maxim (1968) – "start where the learner is at". In considering ISC for an incontinent patient, the nurse should start by seeking his or her understanding of the situation and its management. This enables the nurse to plan how to present the new technique. Further, it is important to assess how the patient feels about changing to a new technique, the level of motivation, capacity to learn, how he or she likes to learn and the degree of support available. The importance of setting an agreed realistic goal with the patient at the outset cannot be understated.

In planning teaching sessions, it is important to adopt a strategy (eg, theory, demonstration, supervised practice) so that the goal can be met. At this stage, the nurse needs to consider involving relatives or significant others in the teaching process if the patient wishes. The plan should include time for the patient to raise concerns, and he or she may find it helpful to meet someone successfully using ISC.

A common mistake is to try to tell the patient everything in one long session. Redman (1981) advises that, in patient teaching, only three major points should be covered in each session. Remember, attention span during illness is even shorter than usual. Major points can be written down for the patient, diagrams can be drawn if useful and the major points should be reiterated in the next session.

Teaching the technique

References (continued)

International Continence Society (1981) Fourth report on the standardisation of terminology of lower urinary tract function. *Brit. Jnl. Urology*, **53**, 333–35.

Lapides, J., Diokro, A.C., Sibler, S.J., Lowe, B.S. (1972) Clean intermittent self-catheterisation in the treatment of urinary tract disease. *Jnl. Urology*, **107**, 459–61.

Murray, K., Lewis, P., Blannin, J., Shepherd, A. (1984) Clean intermittent self-catheterisation in the management of adult lower urinary tract dysfunction. *British Journal of Urology*, **56**, 379–80.

Redman, B.K. (1981) Issues and Concepts in Patient Education. Appleton-Century-Crofts, New York.

Torrens, M.J. (1987) Cystometry. *Hospital Update*, **2**, 11, 1021–29.

Wilson-Barnett, J. (1985) Principles of patient teaching. *Nursing Times*, **81**, 28–29.

Winder, A. (1986) Intermittent self-catheterisation. *The Professional Nurse*, **2**, 2, 58.

Youngjohns, S. (1984) Self-catheterisation. *Journal of District Nursing*, 8–12.

Each session should take place at an appropriate time and in a place where patient and nurse can both relax without disruption. Objectives for the session should be discussed with the patient: for example, the ISC patient needs to begin with a reasonable understanding of the anatomy of the urinary tract and the effects of his or her particular malfunction. Some female patients need help to identify their urethra at first. As the patient progresses in the technique, it is important to give encouragement, correction and praise appropriately. Ample opportunity should be given for the patient to handle the equipment used, to ask questions and to discuss feelings and concerns.

Evaluation of the teaching can be made in many ways. Ask the patient to explain the technique – checking understanding is some measure of your teaching input. Supervision of the patient's attempts is, again, as much a measure of your success as the patient's ability. Achievement of the goals – freedom from infection, happiness and compliance of the patient – are all indicators of your efforts.

ISC will not meet all incontinent patients' needs, and the individual situation of those whose needs it does meet may change over time and make ISC inappropriate; for example, decreasing manual dexterity. However, the technique has significantly improved – and will continue to improve – the quality of life for a body of patients with continence problems. Greater awareness of ISC may help some patients who, as yet, may not have been offered the opportunity.

Catheterisation . . . at your convenience!

A new approach to being continent has been developed which may suit you better than the one you use now. It works better if the type of continence disorder you have means you keep dry between episodes rather than dribble frequently. If you are keen to try and have reasonable use of your hands, this method could help considerably. It is called Intermittent Self-Catheterisation (ISC for short).

What does it involve?

Quite simply, it involves passing a thin tube (catheter) into your bladder between four and six times a day to drain off your urine. It takes about five minutes, and you can do it in the privacy of your own bedroom or bathroom, or in a toilet anywhere. In between times you should remain dry and be able to go about life normally.

ISC is not difficult to learn. The nurse teaching you is willing to discuss your feelings about changing to this way of managing continence, and the catheters you use are available on prescription.

How do you do it?

Slight differences exist in the technique for males and females, but each can manage in 10 simple steps as shown in the boxes below.

Care of your catheter

A catheter can be reused for up to a week and then replaced. After each use, wash it through in running water, shake dry and wipe with a paper towel. Store the catheter dry in a clean washable container.

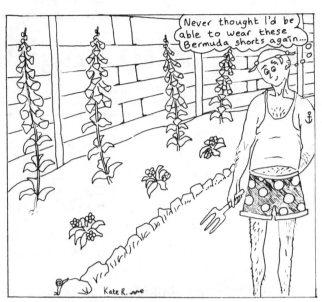

Any other problems?

The risk of infection in your bladder is minimised by keeping to a clean technique and drinking more than two litres a day (about nine cups). If you find you have leakage during sleep, another aid such as pants, a pad or a sheath can be worn at night.

Incontinence during intercourse may be a problem. Restricting your fluids for a couple of hours or self-catheterisation before beginning may bring relief.

If you do have problems, please ring your doctor/ nurse on

. . . .

Female self-catheterisation

1. Assemble your requirements for the procedure.
2. Wash and dry your hands *thoroughly*.
3. Adopt a comfortable position, giving reasonable access to genital area.
4. Spread the labia (lips of the vagina). Wash the opening from front to back with soap and water. Dry gently.
5. Identify the urethral opening. Use a mirror and good light or, if necessary, palpate with finger.
6. Lubricate catheter tip with KY Jelly if necessary. Insert catheter into urethral opening until urine flows.
7. Drain urine into toilet or other container.
8. When urine flow ceases, remove catheter slowly to catch any residue.
9. Wash and dry your catheter and your hands.
10. If your urine smells foul, is cloudy, has persistent presence of blood in it or your catheter becomes painful to pass, contact your nurse or doctor.

Male self-catheterisation

1. Assemble your requirements for the procedure.
2. Wash your penis with soap and water. Dry gently.
3. Wash and dry your hands *thoroughly*.
4. Adopt a comfortable position, giving access to genital area.
5. Lubricate catheter tip with KY Jelly if necessary. It may be necessary to use anaesthetic gel in the urethra instead if the procedure causes pain.
6. Hold your penis fairly tautly. Insert catheter into urethral opening until urine flows.
7. Drain urine into toilet or other container.
8. When urine flow ceases, remove catheter slowly to catch any residue. If urine recommences flowing, stop removing catheter until it ceases.
9. Wash and dry your catheter and your hands.
10. If your urine smells foul, is cloudy, has persistent presence of blood in it or your catheter becomes painful to pass, contact your nurse or doctor.

The pain experienced during an attack of angina can be frightening. However, sufferers can still lead a full life, if they take a few sensible precautions.

Living with angina

Joanne M. Hayward, RGN, BSc(Hons)
Sister, Coronary Care Unit, Norfolk and Norwich Hospital

It is well known that coronary artery disease (CAD) kills or disables many thousands of people each year in Great Britain (WHO, 1985). Now that programmes are underway to prevent heart disease, such as the 'Look After Your Heart' campaign (DHSS, 1987), these figures will hopefully start to decline rapidly. However, vast numbers of people currently suffer from heart disease, particularly angina. Good health education can help them lead as full a life as possible, and the nurse has a vital role in this (Edwards, 1987).

Inadequate blood supply

References

Blackburn, H. (1983) Physical activity and coronary heart disease: a brief update and population view. *Journal of Cardiac Rehabilitation,* **3,** 101-111.

Department of Health and Social Security, Health Education Authority (1987) Look after your heart: a campaign to encourage healthier lifestyles in England. DHSS, London.

Edwards, J. (1987) Controlling a killer. *Nursing Times,* **83,** 15, 27-8.

Fogarty, A., Hills, S., Sloan, C., (1986) Finding the facts on glyceryl trinitrate tablets. *Nursing Times,* **82,** 35, 38-9.

Julian, D.G. (1983) Cardiology. (4th Edn.) Bailliere Tindall,

Mulcahy, R. (1983) Influence of cigarette smoking on morbity and mortality after myocardial infarction. *British Heart Journal,* **49,** 410-415.

Patel, C. (1985) Trial of relaxation in reducing coronary risk: four year follow-up. *British Medical Journal,* **290,** 6475, 1103-6.

World Health Organisation (1982) Expert committee report on the prevention of coronary disease. Technical Report Series No. 678. WHO, Geneva.

World Health Organisation (1985) World Statistics Quarterly, 38-2. WHO, Geneva.

Reducing the risk

Angina occurs when the coronary arteries are unable to supply adequate blood and/or oxygen to the myocardium of the heart. This may be the result of a decrease in the supply of oxygen or an increase in the demands of the heart. Most patients have narrowing or blocking of their coronary arteries due to atheroma, therefore, when the heart's demand for oxygen increases, for example with exertion or stress, these needs cannot be met as a greater blood flow through the arteries cannot be achieved. This results in ischaemia which causes the chest pain or discomfort of angina. If the blockage of the arteries is complete and ischaemia persists, myocardial infarction may occur. Angina may be seen as a warning that the heart muscle is not receiving enough oxygen and that the situation must be improved to prevent a myocardial infarction, with its potentially fatal consequences.

Angina translates from the Latin as 'strangling of the chest', reflected in its description by patients as burning, crushing, squeezing or heaviness in the centre of the chest. It may radiate to the neck, arms, elbows or jaw, most typically on the left side. It is exacerbated by anything which will increase the demand of the heart for oxygen or reduce its supply, for example, exercise, emotion, tachycardia or anaemia, though in some cases it may occur spontaneously. It is usually relieved by rest, oxygen and nitrates, such as sublingual glyceryl trinitrate (GTN).

The diagnosis of angina may seem particularly devastating to the patient, given the heart's function in maintaining life and also its image as the centre of emotions (Julian, 1983). They will need help and support in coming to terms with and understanding their diagnosis.

The World Health Organisation (1982) has recommended that people take measures to reduce the risk of CAD, including reducing consumption of saturated fats and cholesterol, getting treatment for high blood pressure, stopping smoking and increasing exercise. These are most effective when started at a young age but can also help patients with CAD: giving up smoking after a myocardial infarction can halve the risk of it recurring (Mulcahy, 1983). The benefits of exercise (Blackburn, 1983) and relaxation (Patel, 1985) have also been shown.

Patients also need to understand their medication to use it effectively. Many patients do not know how to use or store their GTN correctly (Fogarty et al, 1986) this may result in the tablets becoming ineffective, causing unnecessary suffering and morbidity. The handout opposite gives guidelines on living with angina, to help patients lead as normal a life as possible and reduce the risk of myocardial infarction.

Living With Angina

What is angina?

Angina occurs when the blood flow to your heart is decreased, so not enough oxygen reaches the heart muscle. This is usually due to a build-up of 'fatty plugs' in the arteries, which block the flow of the blood (Figure 1).

While you are resting the blood supply to the heart is usually sufficient. However, if you exercise or increase the heart's need for oxygen in other ways (Table 1), this extra need cannot be met and a 'cramp' results in the heart muscle. You may feel this as pain or tightness in the chest and often in the left arm or jaw as well, or it may only be felt in the arm or jaw – everyone's pain is individual.

Angina is a warning signal that the heart is not getting enough oxygen and something must be done to prevent any damage occuring.

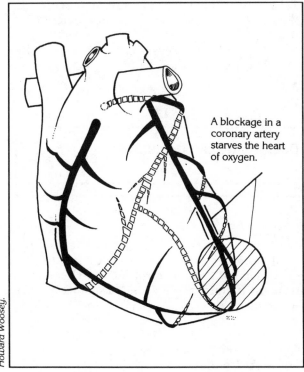

A blockage in a coronary artery starves the heart of oxygen.

Howard Woosey.

Figure 1. The heart and its coronary arteries.

What you can do to help yourself

Smoking   It is essential that you stop at once. Smoking increases the 'clogging' of the blood vessels. Do seek help from your doctor or a local support group if you need it. Try to persuade the rest of the family to give up with you. It's easier together.

Temperatures   Try to avoid extremes of hot and cold. Make sure that you wrap up well if you do have to go out in cold weather and avoid going on holiday to places that you know are going to be very hot.

- Exercise or exertion.
- Extremes of temperature.
- Emotion or stress.
- A heavy meal.
- Sexual activity.

Try to identify those things which cause your angina and consider how these could be changed or avoided.

Table 1. Things that may increase the heart's demand for oxygen.

Exercise   This will help to strengthen the heart, but you should not try to do activities which provoke your chest pain. A short walk at a gentle pace each day will help.

Relaxation   Try to avoid any activity which may be stressful to you, such as particular work situations or arguments. Find some time to rest every day and try taking up a relaxing hobby which will take your mind off any worries you may have.

Sexual activity   This needs not be avoided, but it may help to take a more passive role to lessen the exertion on your heart. Try taking Glyceryl trinitrate (GTN) just beforehand if sexual activity normally provokes your chest pain.

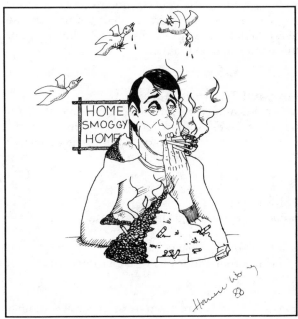

Smoking increases the clogging of the arteries.

Diet If you are overweight, get advice on how to lose weight. The less weight the body has to carry the less work the heart has to do. In general, try to avoid fatty or fried food and try changing to a low fat margarine and skimmed milk. A high fibre diet is also good for your general health. You should also try to cut down on salt in your food as this can cause high blood pressure.

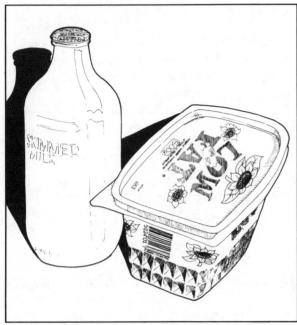

Try changing to a low fat margarine and skimmed milk.

Your medications

You may be given a variety of tablets for your angina, for specific information on each, please ask your nurse or doctor. It is important that you take your tablets regularly as prescribed, try to establish a routine where you take your tablets at the same times each day to help you to remember them. Always make sure you do not run out of your supplies and ask for more in plenty of time. Some heart tablets may cause headaches initially but these will subside in time.

Glyceryl Trinitrate (GTN)
This medication comes as a tablet or spray and is for use in the event of an angina attack. Some simple rules should be followed to ensure you get effective relief:

Tablets
● Place one under the tongue and allow to dissolve.

● If the tablets cause headaches it may help to spit out the remainder of the tablet once your pain has gone.

● Always store correctly in the dark glass container supplied, with no cotton wool.

● Discard remaining tablets eight weeks after opening and obtain a fresh supply.

● Carry your tablets with you at all times.

GTN Spray
● No need to shake.

● Spray 1-2 times under the tongue, taking care not to breathe and blow away the spray.

● Carry your spray with you at all times.

● Spray will last until empty.

If you have an angina attack
● Stop and rest.

● Take your GTN tablets or spray. If your pain is not relieved by the first dose this should be repeated.
  If your pain is very severe or is not relieved by GTN contact your doctor, as further help may be needed.

Doctor's telephone number

....

If your pain increases in frequency or severity, consult your doctor as it may be necessary to alter your tablets for better control. Advice should also be sought if you start to experience angina while you are resting.

Useful address:-
The British Heart Foundation,
102 Gloucester Place, London, W1H 4DH.

The Foundation provides a range of booklets and information on many aspects of heart disease including 'What is Angina' and 'Diet and Your Heart'.

Remember

Your angina is a warning that you need to take more care of your heart.

If you follow the advice given here, you will reduce the strain on your heart.

The patient's own skills in catheter management will make all the difference to their confidence and health at home. Careful teaching of newly catheterised patients will support them in developing these skills and with them their independence.

Teaching patients to cope with catheters at home

Elizabeth Wright, SRN, DipN
Ward Sister, Male Surgical Ward, The Middlesex Hospital, London

An important part of the nurse's role is that of a health educator and promoter of independence in patients' self-care. This is particularly true when preparing patients to cope at home with their catheter drainage system.

The promotion of the patients' independence in catheter care, whenever possible is likely to reduce the risks of cross infection (Gould, 1985). Gould found that only 10 wards in her study of 19 had developed a policy of encouraging patients to take on responsibility for their own catheter care, and only 11 wards provided information regarding catheter management for patients and their relatives.

The onus lies firmly with the nurse to educate patients and their relatives about their catheter drainage system and how to help prevent infection entering the system. The promotion of self-care is particularly relevant in preventing cross infection in these patients.

Guidelines for management

Nurses are coming to terms with their role as health educators, and to assist the nurses on my ward with this unfamiliar role, I decided to compile a list of basic guidelines for catheter management. This was discussed with the relevant consultant medical staff and infection control sister, before being issued to both patients and staff. It is not intended to replace the information given in procedure manuals within the health authority, but to offer brief basic information on catheter management.

The list of guidelines for patients and staff offer relevant information to each group. For instance, patients require advice to be written in a more informal format, whereas nursing staff require facts and technical details of care based on research.

Nursing guidelines

1. Catheterisation should be performed as an aseptic procedure. Use the smallest size possible to reduce bladder neck irritation and leaking of urine. Consider also whether the patient will require a long term catheter. Document the type and size of catheter used and the amount of water required to inflate the balloon.

2. The patient should drink at least 1-2 litres every day of any fluid, (tea, coffee or milk may be more palatable than water for instance.) This only applies to patients with normal renal function.

3. Support the catheter bag on a stand and ensure the outlet tap is not in contact with the floor.

4. Do not raise the catheter drainage bag above the level of the patient's bladder for any length of time.

5. Teach the patient meatal cleansing, using an Inco-wipe and soap and water. Ensure that the foreskin is replaced, after the glans has been cleaned to prevent paraphimosis. Hands should be washed before and after this technique.

6. Empty the outlet tap using gloves (wash hands also before and after procedure) using the patient's individual jug, and ensuring the tap does not touch the sides. Wipe the tap with an alcohol impregnated wipe afterwards. If the patient does this, he or she must also wash hands before and after the procedure.

7. Observe the colour of the urine; it should not be cloudy, dark in colour or offensive to smell. If the patient develops a pyrexia, becomes confused, has a rigor, or has cloudy, offensive urine, it may indicate a urinary tract infection and a specimen should be obtained for culture. Urine cultures should also be routinely obtained every week.

8. Do not routinely disconnect the catheter from the drainage bag, unless the bag is faulty, blocked with clots or debris, or the patient requires a bladder washout. Disconnection should be documented and reported to the nurse in charge.

9. If possible put catheterised and non catheterised patients in adjacent beds.

10. Do not allow the catheter or drainage bag to kink or obstruct the urine flow.

The patient guidelines in the handout on page 99 can be photocopied for distribution to catheterised patients who are being discharged with their catheter still in situ.

Your Guide to Catheter Care

Your urethral catheter

The tube that you have, (or will have) in place, drains urine from the bladder. It is there because you are either unable to pass your urine sufficiently well yourself, due to a blockage to your bladder, or you have had surgery that still needs time to heal inside. The tube is called a catheter, and it is held in place by a balloon that stops it from falling out of your bladder.

The catheter drains urine into a bag that you can either carry or attach to your leg, and can be emptied from a tap at the base of the bags. The picture below shows you the position of the catheter and how it works.

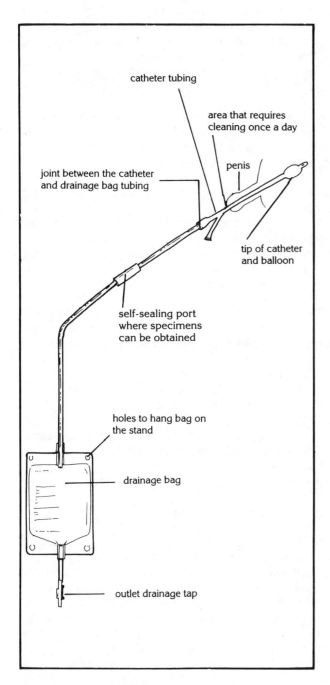

Your catheter drainage system.

If catheters are not looked after properly, they can cause urinary infections. This guide explains how you can help prevent this from happening. If you do not understand anything, or you have any problems or worries concerning your catheter, contact either the sister or staff nurse on the ward you were treated or the district nurse, who will be able to help you.

1. Do not disconnect the catheter from the drainage bag unless it is absolutely necessary, to prevent infection entering the system. If it does get disconnected, inform the district nurse.

2. You should drink at least 12-14 cups (1-2 litres) of any kind of fluid you wish eg, tea, coffee or milk. This will help the urine to flow more easily, and prevent infections occurring in the urine.

3. Your urine should be pale yellow in colour. If there is debris in it, or it is dark yellow in colour with an offensive smell, you may have an infection and need to drink more. You should also visit your general practitioner to give him a specimen of urine so he can determine if you do have an infection present.

4. The drainage bag should always be lower than the level of your pelvis, on a stand or fixed to your leg or around your waist. Do not put it in your dressing gown pocket or leave it lying on the floor or anywhere else.

You can bath or shower with the catheter in place, but be careful not to pull it unnecessarily or hang it on the side of the bath or shower. Please clean around the site where the catheter enters your body at least once a day to keep it clean. Use cotton wool Inco-wipe for this purpose and soap and water (luke warm). If you have any unusual offensive discharge, report it to your district nurse or general practitioner.

6. Eat plenty of wholemeal bread or bran, fruit and vegetables to prevent constipation.

7. Do not allow the catheter tube to kink, as this will prevent the drainage of urine, which may then leak around the outside of the catheter. Leakage of urine around the catheter may also indicate that the bladder is irritated by the catheter; contact your general practitioner or the ward staff who will be able to advise you.

8. If the catheter falls out or you are concerned about any problems related to it, please contact the ward staff and speak to the sister or staff nurse or contact the district nurse.

Telephone number: ....

Asthma is one of the most common chronic diseases in the UK. If sufferers are aware of the causes of their attacks they can do much to control their condition, yet research shows that they are often given little information about it.

Living with asthma

Gill A. Hek, RGN, NDN, CertEd(FE)
Nurse Tutor, Avon College of Nursing and Midwifery, Bristol

Asthma is one of the most common chronic diseases seen in general practice. A general practice population of 2,500 will contain about 125 patients who suffer from it in varying degrees (Clark and Rees, 1985). It is defined as 'widespread airways obstruction which is reversible over short periods of time, either spontaneously or as a result of treatment.'

Boys suffer from asthma two to three times more frequently than girls, but by adulthood the prevalence is the same. Up to the age of 10, new cases are frequent, then prevalence drops, with another increase of new cases at around the age of 40 years. 50 per cent of child sufferers will grow out of the condition.

In Britain there are around 2,000 deaths from asthma every year, and in many sufferers there is significant morbidity, producing loss of time from work and school, and disruption to normal family activities. There are many precipitating factors (Table 1), some impossible to avoid.

The reactive airways of a patient with asthma are provoked by many 'trigger factors'. These include:-	
Pollens	Occupational dusts
House dust mites	and chemicals
Animals	Psychological
Infection	factors
Exercise	Menstruation
Dust	Pregnancy
Pollution	Gastro-
Foods	oesophageal
Drugs	reflux
Fungi	Thyroid disease

Table 1. Precipitating factors in asthma.

Symptoms

Breathlessness is usually the main symptom of asthma. Breathing out is usually more difficult than breathing in.

Wheezing is a result of the effort to breathe out, and is due to the narrowing of the airways.

Cough is a common accompaniment to the breathlessness and wheezing, especially in children, indeed in some children, coughing, especially at night, may be the only sign of asthma.

Caring for people with asthma

Reference
Clark, T. and Rees, J. (1985). Practical Management of Asthma. Martin Dunitz, London.

Bibliography
Allen and Hanbury Ltd (1985)
Understanding Asthma. Leaflet produced by Allen and Hanbury Ltd.
Lane, D.J. and Storr, A. (1979) Asthma, The Facts. Oxford University Press, Oxford.
Clark, T. and Rees, J. (1985) Practical Management of Asthma. Martin Dunitz, London.
This is essential reading for nurses caring for people with asthma.

Useful information
Leaflets and information regarding correct use of inhalers is available from:- Local Chemists
Health Education Departments
Drug companies, eg Allen and Hanburys, Fisons Plc
The Asthma Society, 300 Upper Street, London N1 2XX.
Most leaflets are free and are an essential requirement for anyone involved to a great extent with asthmatic patients.

Nurses caring for asthmatic patients need to be knowledgeable about the condition, and must be effective when educating asthmatic patients about its management. The areas nurses should be familiar with include:

- How to use a peak flow meter to good effect and how to determine an individual's peak expiratory flow rate.
- The common drugs used to control asthma, their regimens and which drugs should be used on a patient having an attack.
- The side effects and overdosage of the common drugs.
- How to use inhalers, rotahalers, spinhalers, diskhalers, turbohalers, 'spacer devices' and nebulisers to good effect.
- How to tell when a patient's condition is worsening.
- What to do when a patient has an attack, and how to tell whether it is being controlled.

Even if psychological factors precipitated an asthma attack, the response is physiological and the same treatments as for other 'trigger' factors must be given. Asthma attacks are extremely stressful to patient and family. By creating a relaxed atmosphere, being confident in their approach and giving effective advice to the family, nurses can do much to relieve anxiety.

There is a lot of research suggesting that people with asthma are not educated effectively regarding their condition. Nurses are in an excellent position to change this by educating them in the community, following the common, well established methods of treatment. This may mean as little as checking a patient's inhaler technique, and advising as necessary, or it may require detailed explanation of the condition and how best to control it.

The handout opposite can be photocopied and distributed freely.

Living with Asthma

This handout explains about asthma and how to control it. Keep it handy, with your doctor's phone number, so you can use it to help you when you have an attack.

Doctor's phone number . . . .

What is asthma?

In an asthma attack the tubes to the lungs become too narrow. It's like trying to breathe through a straw when you are used to a hosepipe. The things that you might notice are:-
- Wheezing
- Tight chest
- Shortness of breath
- Cough
- Yellow sticky phlegm

For most people, everything will return to normal either on its own or by taking medication. There are two main types of medication for people who have asthma, and you may be taking one or both types.

Drugs for preventing asthma

Your doctor may prescribe some drugs for you to take regularly to help stop you getting attacks. They will have to be taken every day, sometimes three or four times, depending on what the doctor has told you. Some common medicines are:-
- Intal
- Becotide
- Pulmicort
- Becloforte

Drugs for opening up the airways

These medicines, often in the form of an inhaler are called **Bronchodilators.** They work by opening up the airways when you are having an attack.
Some common bronchodilators are:-
- Ventolin
- Atrovent
- Bricanyl
- Theophylline, eg Phyllocontin
  Neulin
  Uniphyllin

Sometimes the doctor may prescribe a course of steroids for you after a bad attack. When the asthma is back under control, you will not normally need to take these powerful drugs.

Recognising an attack

You must learn to recognise when an attack might occur, or when your asthma is not properly under control, by assessing the signs. Any of the following signs might suggest that the asthma is not in total control, and you will need to seek advice.
- Your normal medication is not working as well as it used to.
- You wake up in the morning coughing, wheezing or with a tight chest.
- You are waking up in the night with coughing and/or wheezing.
- You find that you are short of breath at the beginning of the day.
- Peak flow readings are lower than usual.
- You can't take exercise without getting symptoms.

During an attack

Keep calm and as relaxed as possible. Concentrate on taking your medication correctly.
It may help to sit upright with your shoulders forward, leaning on a high table. It may be more comfortable to lean on a pillow (Figure 1).
A steamy kettle in the room may help to loosen the phlegm on your chest.

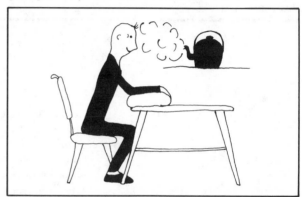

Figure 1. Sit upright with your shoulders forward.

If you are suffering any of the following symptoms, then you must seek help immediately from your doctor or hospital:
- Blueness around the lips.
- Difficulty in speaking.
- Breathlessness when resting.
- Fast pulse.
- Peak flow reading below 100 l/min.

Remember

You must know exactly how to take your medicines, and the correct way to use the inhalers. If you are unsure, your doctor, practice nurse, or chemist will show you how it is done.

Asthma is not 'all in the mind'. You must find out what starts your asthma off, and try hard to avoid it again.

Exercise, especially swimming is very good for asthma sufferers. If you are worried about swimming, ask your doctor.

Useful address

The Asthma Society,
300 Upper Street,
London N1 2XX.

The Asthma Society supply leaflets and information on the correct use of inhalers. These are also available from chemists.

Coeliac disease is a distressing chronic disease that affects the long term health and growth of small children. There is no known cure, but the symptoms can be completely relieved by removing all foods containing gluten from the diet. One in fifteen hundred people have coeliac disease and if they are to be able to enjoy their food while still preventing their symptoms, it is important that they have access to as many foods as possible, and also to current advice as to what is available.

Gluten-free diets — helping patients to cope

Myra Ibbotson, PhD, BSc, SRD
Freelance Dietitian

Coeliac disease is a malabsorption syndrome caused by an idiosyncracy in the way the digestive tract handles gluten, part of the protein fraction of wheat. Gluten is composed of two proteins, gliadin and glutenin. Gliadin is the 'toxic' fraction which causes coeliac disease by interfering with the normal uptake of nutrients by the mucosa of the small intestine. The mucosal cells become flat instead of columnar and lose their villi, resulting in a much smaller surface area for absorption. The reasons for the occurrence of coeliac disease are still not fully known.

Impaired absorption

Coeliac disease results in the impaired absorption of a wide range of nutrients; fat malabsorption leads to steatorrhoea: the stools are large, pale, offensive and difficult to flush away (because of their high fat content). Vitamin, mineral, carbohydrate and protein absorption are also affected (Ward, 1982).

Patients usually present in early childhood (before three years), generally at the time of weaning, when foods containing wheat are given. The change in the nature of the stool, and the pale, pot bellied appearance and failure to thrive are characteristic diagnostic features. Coeliac disease can also develop in adults, when steatorrhoea and loss of appetite are the common features. Diagnosis is confirmed when a jejunal biopsy reveals the characteristically flattened mucosa.

Iron and folate preparations

Anaemia is often present, resulting from the poor uptake of iron, a low serum folate level is common, although megaloblastic anaemia as a result of this is usually seen only in adult cases. As absorption improves on a gluten-free diet, nutritional problems such as these anaemias are automatically resolved. Iron and folate preparations are given in the short term until the recovery of the gut mucosa is complete (Ward, 1982).

The symptoms can be relieved and normal growth is re-established in children by removing gluten from the diet; effectively by avoiding wheat although most people with coeliac disease are also advised to avoid rye, barley and oats.

Avoiding the stigma

Children in groups (for example, at school) are quick to spot and to stigmatise any member of the group who is different in some way. A child with coeliac disease may be singled out and victimised and could be treated as the 'odd man out' at home, too. These potential problems can be minimised by sensitive discussion with the child's family. Packed lunches will avoid the problems which may be presented by school meals, and once the child has learnt which foods to avoid, he or she will be able to make the correct choices at parties and other situations involving meals away from home (Henry, 1980).

Planning the diet

It may seem an impossible task to completely exclude wheat and its products from the diet, but this is becoming much simpler as manufacturers become more willing to label foods appropriately (the gluten-free symbol is shown below) and as manufacturers of gluten-free products become more adventurous. A variety of gluten-free pastas are now available, for example, as well as choc chip cookies, and a high fibre loaf that looks just like a normal brown loaf (an important consideration for a child taking packed lunches to school). The "high fibre" component, incidentally, may be rice bran, sugar beet pulp or pea flour.

Patients can be encouraged to try any recipe they like, providing they use the appropriate gluten-free substitutes where necessary. The most successful recipes will be those where the unique structural qualities of gluten are not needed. Recipes where a soft texture (eg. sponge cakes) or a "short" texture (eg. shortcake biscuits) are desirable are very successful.

Cornflour can be used for thickening sauces and gravies, and finely crushed cornflakes make a crisp "breadcrumb" coating for fish or meat. A few recipe suggestions have been given on the handout but patients should be encouraged to experiment for themselves.

The Coeliac Society

The gluten-free diet is a strict lifelong diet for someone with coeliac disease. The Coeliac Society can provide support in the form of local group meetings, a newsletter and a regularly updated list of manufactured products free from gluten. Patients should be encouraged to join. They can be contacted by writing to the Coeliac Society, PO Box 181, London NW2 2QY.

Certain gluten-free products, such as bread or bread mixes, flour and plain biscuits are prescribable on form FP10, endorsed ACBS (Advisory Committee on Borderline Substances).

Dermatitis herpetiformis

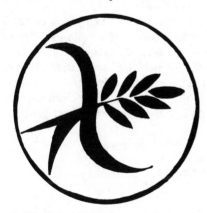

The gluten-free symbol or "crossed grained"

A gluten-free diet may also be prescribed for dermatitis herpetiformis, an itchy skin rash with raised, reddened spots particularly on elbows, shoulders and knees, although it can occur anywhere. In about 60 to 75 per cent of patients, there is also small intestinal damage similar to coeliac disease. Treatment for dermatitis herpetiformis is not, however, straightforward, and each case must be treated individually. There is still a lot of controversy about the usefulness of a gluten-free diet in this condition.

References
Henry, C.L. (1980) A patient's view of a gluten-free diet. *Journal of Human Nutrition* **34** 50. J. Libby and Co. (London)
Ward, R. (1982) Coeliac disease. *Nutrition and Food Science.* March/April 1982 10-12. Haymarket Publishing (London)

Bibliography
Rawcliff, P. and Rolph, R. The Gluten Free Diet Book, (1985) Durnitz. A very helpful guide for sufferers and their families.

The handout overleaf can be photocopied and distributed to patients and their families, but it is advisable to first refer to the dietitian involved.

Living With a Gluten-Free Diet

This handout will provide you with some advice and ideas for planning a gluten-free diet. More help is available from your dietitian and your district nurse of health visitor. Do not hesitate to contact them if you are worried about any aspect of your diet or your health and always consult your dietitian regularly.

Useful address

To keep up to date with the latest gluten-free ideas and recipes, join the Coeliac Society. Send a stamped addressed envelope to:
The Coeliac Society, PO Box 200, High Wycombe, Bucks, HP11 2HY.

The services of the Society are only available to people with clinically diagnosed coelic disease or dermatitis herpetiformis. Their list of Gluten-Free Manufactured Products is published annually in April and is automatically sent to members. It is also updated monthly on BBC Ceefax, page 256.

Members also receive The Crossed Grain, a twice yearly magazine and the Society also publish a handbook, a video and information on travel and holidays.

Recipe ideas

The two recipes below are simply examples to show that a gluten-free diet does not mean you cannot eat foods that usually contain wheat products. Ask your dietitian to recommend a gluten-free recipe book and try some experiments of your own when you are used to using the new ingredients.

Gluten-free biscuits (makes about 25-30)
100g (4oz) gluten-free flour
100g (4oz) butter or margarine
75g (3oz) caster sugar
2 teaspoons gluten-free baking powder
1 egg, lightly beaten
vanilla essence or other flavouring as desired
Preheat oven to 350 deg F, 180 deg C, gas mark 4.
Cream fat and sugar together, sift together flour and baking powder and stir into creamed mixture. Add one or two drops of vanilla essence or chosen flavouring. Mix in the egg and roll out, using gluten-free flour to dust surfaces and rolling pin, to about ¼ inch thickness, then cut into shapes. Bake on a greased baking sheet for 15-20 minutes.
Alternative flavourings include 1oz finely chopped glacé cherries, 1oz dried fruit, 2oz dessicated coconut, or 2 teaspoons powdered ginger.

Sponge cake
150g (6oz) gluten-free flour
150g (6oz) Margarine (at room temperature)
150g (6oz) caster sugar
1 teaspoon gluten-free baking powder
3 eggs
grated rind of one lemon/orange or a few drops of vanilla essence
Preheat the oven to 355 deg F, 190 deg C, gas mark 5. Put all ingredients into a bowl and mix for 1-2 minutes with an electric mixer or 2-3 minutes by hand.
Pour mixture into a greased 7 inch sponge tin and bake for 20-25 minutes. Cool on a rack then split and sandwich with jam, buttercream or fruit and whipped cream as desired.

The "crossed grain" symbol. This tells you that food products are gluten-free.

Foods to eat and avoid on a gluten-free diet

FOODS ALLOWED	FOODS NOT ALLOWED
Cereals: Rice, maize, (sweetcorn, cornflour) gluten-free pasta and flour, arrowroot, potato flour, soya, flour, pea flour, rice flour Sago, tapioca Soya or rice bran Gluten-free bread, cakes or biscuits Cornflakes, Rice Krispies	**Cereals:** Wheat, barley, rye, oats Ordinary pasta (spaghetti, macaroni) ordinary flour Semolina Wheat germ wheat bran Ordinary bread, cakes or biscuits Starch reduced bread, crispbreads Weetabix, bran type cereals, Grapenuts, puffed wheat, muesli, Shredded wheat and all other wheat based cereals
Meat: All fresh/frozen meat	**Meat:** Sausages*, pies* sausage rolls*, beefburgers*, meat paste*, pate*
Fish: All varieties, fresh or frozen	**Fish:** Bread crumbed or battered fish, fish in sauce
Cheese: All whole cheeses	**Cheese:** Some cheese spreads
Eggs: Hen or duck	
Milk: Fresh, evaporated, dried, skimmed, condensed, cream, sour cream, yogurt (check the label).	**Milk:** Synthetic cream*
Fruit: All kinds, fresh, tinned, juice or frozen	**Fruit:** Fruit pie fillings*
Vegetables: All kinds, fresh, tinned or frozen	**Vegetables:** Baked beans*, instant potato*, potato/vegetable salad with salad cream type dressing*
Nuts: All kinds except dry roasted peanuts	**Nuts:** Dry roasted peanuts
Beverages: Tea, coffee, cocoa, soda, water, squashes, fizzy drinks	**Beverages:** Bengers, Horlicks, barley water, vending machine drinks*
Alcoholic drinks: Most pub beers, wines and spirits, liqueurs and fortified wines	**Alcoholic drinks:** Home brewed or 'real ales'
Fats: Oil, butter, margarine, lard, dripping	**Fats:** Packet suet*
Sugars and Preserves: Jam, marmalade, honey	**Sugars and Preserves:** Lemon curd, mincemeat, chocolate
Seasonings: Salt, freshly ground pepper, herbs, spices, vinegar, Bovril, Marmite	**Seasonings:** Curry powder*, stock cubes*, sauces, chutneys, pickles
Miscellaneous: Yeast, cream of tartar, bicarbonate of soda	**Miscellaneous:** Baking powder

Foods in the 'not allowed' column marked * have certain gluten-free formulations available. Your dietitian will tell you where to get them.

Your patient needs to know and understand about his medication. By explaining and demonstrating clearly to him, you can make sure that his treatment continues effectively after discharge.

Medication to take home

Janet Gooch, SRN, DipN(Lond) RCNT
Ward Sister, Brighton General Hospital

Few patients are, as yet, allowed to control their own medication in hospital and yet they are expected to do so correctly on discharge. A written reminder can be a useful means of ensuring that the patient is given sufficient knowledge to make that possible.

Lack of knowledge

Frequently patients bring drugs into hospital but have little knowledge of why they are taking them. Rarely can they state the action of the drugs, their side effects, or the length of time they are to be taken. It is not rare for them to admit to having stopped taking a drug for some personal reason and be unaware of whether this is important or not. Apart from the danger of such a lack of knowledge there are great financial implications — drugs taken for too long and those wasted are an expense to the Health Service that we cannot afford.

Most patients take drugs given to them by nurses without question, merely because they are prescribed by the doctor. Maybe they *should* ask if they want to know what the drug is for, but they have to contend with the myth of the busy nurse. It takes great courage to delay trained nurses long enough to query each tablet or draught. The onus has to be on the nurses to supply the necessary information.

A hospital admission is an opportunity to educate patients about their drugs, and it should not be missed.

Information needed

Terminology The terminology used when teaching about drugs should suit each individual patient to whom the information is given. Few require explanation of the full biological action of their tablets but everyone needs to know in their own terms why they are taking something.

Side effects If nurses are aware of side effects of any drug given to a patient it should be possible to make him aware of these without causing such concern that he decides not to take the medicine.

Time Limits If there is a finite period set by the prescription then the patient should know this. Where life-long prescriptions are expected then equally the patient must be made aware that this essential medication should not be stopped without consulting a doctor. Where there is doubt about the time limit the patient can be told to ask regularly about this.

Questions The more we can encourage patients to question (and learn to understand) their own health care, with both doctors and nurses, the better they will be equipped to comply with our requirements.

Special points

● The safety tops on bottles of tablets were designed to prevent children opening them — in practice they defeat the elderly more than the young. Does the patient know how to remove the top? Are his hands capable of the necessary manipulation? If not, the pharmacist can provide alternative containers if requested.
● The print on the bottle labels is rather small. Can the patient discern the words? Can he in fact read?

- Many people are unaware of expiry dates on medicines and tablets. When given drugs to take home does the patient know if such an expiry time exists on any of them?
- Is this an opportunity to remind patients to get rid of all the old drugs they may have at home? Do they know about drug safety?

A written plan of medications to be taken at home can be completed with the patient and given to him to take away with the drugs. A suggested format and a completed example follow. The symbols can be used to explain to patients who cannot read — a symbol on the bottle would also appear on the chart as illustrated.

The outline plan below may be photocopied for distribution to patients.

PATIENT'S NAME: –									
NAME OF DRUG AND ITS ACTION	BREAK-FAST TIME	WHEN TO TAKE THE DRUG						WHEN TO STOP TAKING THE DRUG	SPECIAL POINTS
		LUNCH TIME	TEA TIME	SUPPER TIME	BED TIME				
DIGOXIN to regulate heart beats	ONE TABLET							ONLY WHEN YOUR DOCTOR SAYS SO CHECK EACH TIME YOU SEE HIM	
FERROUS SULPHATE Iron tablets for your anaemia	TWO TABLETS			TWO TABLETS				ON 5/12/85	THIS WILL MAKE YOUR MOTIONS BLACK. THAT IS NORMAL
MILPAR For your bowels	ONE SPOONFUL				ONE SPOONFUL			ASK WHEN YOU COME TO OUTPATIENTS	
NAVIDREX K To make you pass more water and stop ankle swelling	ONE TABLET							ONLY WHEN YOUR DOCTOR SAYS SO -CHECK WHEN YOU SEE HIM NEXT MONTH	SWALLOW WHOLE DO NOT CHEW

PATIENT'S NAME: –									
NAME OF DRUG AND ITS ACTION	BREAK-FAST TIME	WHEN TO TAKE THE DRUG						WHEN TO STOP TAKING THE DRUG	SPECIAL POINTS
		LUNCH TIME	TEA TIME	SUPPER TIME	BED TIME				

Patients going home with an indwelling catheter need to know how to cope with it correctly if complications are to be avoided. These information sheets may help them to do so.

Care of the catheter at home

Janet Gooch, SRN, DipN(Lond), RCNT
Ward Sister, Brighton General Hospital

Equipment

There is a wide choice of appliance available from which each patient can select the one most suited to his needs and life style. Several methods may be tried in the hospital ward before the final selection is made. If this choice later proves to be less successful than imagined then it is possible to ask for a known alternative.

Explanation

To know how to manage the catheter and drainage system correctly, and to minimize the risk of infection, it is necessary to understand how the system works and how problems could arise.

1. Urine is made by the kidneys and is normally stored in the bladder until you are ready to go to the toilet to pass the water. The catheter is a tube that is put into the bladder and kept there by a small balloon on its end. In this way the urine passes directly into the drainage bag attached to the catheter instead of remaining in the bladder. Ask your nurse if you are unsure of the reason for your catheter.
2. As long as the catheter and tubing are free of kinks or loops, and the bag is kept below the end of the catheter, there will be a free passage of urine. Interruption of this free flow can cause a "damming up" of urine which could increase the risk of infection.
3. Pulling on the catheter makes the balloon rub on the inside of the bladder and causes soreness.
4. Infection in the drainage system could come from dirty hands and from the area around the catheter where bacteria multiply if they are not removed by washing. It is therefore essential to wash the hands with soap and water before and after handling any part of the catheter, tubing, or bag. The area around the catheter needs washing at least once a day and after each bowel action — this washing should be from front to back so that bacteria from the back passage are not brought forward around the catheter.
5. A flow of urine washing down the inside of the tubing helps to keep the tube clean. To maintain a steady flow it is necessary to drink plenty of fluids to make the urine. It is better to drink small amounts regularly throughout the day rather than large amounts just once or twice.
6. Constipation can cause pressure on the catheter and block the flow of urine.

Other points

- People at home generally have divan type beds that are unsuitable for the bedside hanger used in hospital. A floor-standing hanger supplied for use at night avoids lying the drainage bag on the floor.
- Painful spasms of the bladder sometimes occur when the catheter is first inserted. These are explained by the reaction of the body to the strange tube and stop once this is overcome. If they should recur it may be because the tube is blocked and help is needed to deal with this. In this case, your community nurse should be contacted.
- Very occasionally some bleeding occurs through or around a catheter. Unless you have been told to expect this, such bleeding should always be reported to your doctor.
- Remember that catheter bags (for both day and night use) are available on prescription.

These information sheets may be photocopied for distribution to patients.

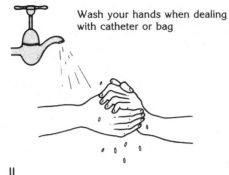

Wash your hands when dealing with catheter or bag

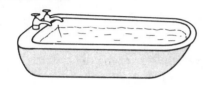

A daily shower or bath helps keep the area around the catheter clean

Drink at least 4 pints of fluid every day

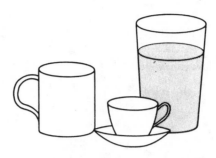

Fresh fruit, bran, cereals, and wholemeal bread help avoid constipation

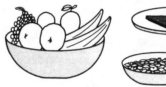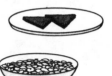

Make sure the catheter and tubing are free of kinks

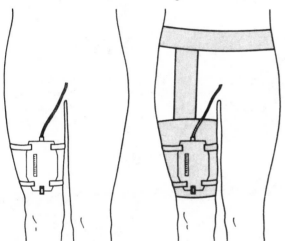

During the day

Rinse the night bag with warm water and hang it up to dry during the day

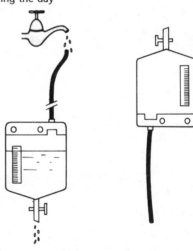

Use a new night bag every few days when the old one deteriorates

And at night

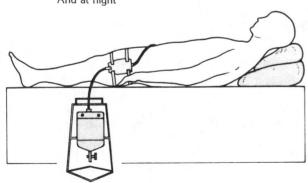

When to seek help
- If no urine drains into the bag
- If the urine leaks round the catheter
- If the urine becomes thick and cloudy
- If the urine becomes smelly
- If the catheter feels "gritty" when rolled between your fingers
- If any bleeding occurs
- If you are worried